1472

Physician's Guide
to Sunscreens

Physician's Guide to Sunscreens

edited by

NICHOLAS J. LOWE

Skin Research Foundation of California
Santa Monica, California

UCLA School of Medicine
Los Angeles, California

MARCEL DEKKER, INC.   **New York • Basel • Hong Kong**

Library of Congress Cataloging-in-Publication Data

Physician's guide to sunscreens / edited by Nicholas J. Lowe.
   p. cm.
    The contents of this volume were originally published in
Sunscreens: development, evaluation, and regulatory aspects, edited
by N.J. Lowe and N.A. Shaath. c 1990 by Marcel Dekker, Inc.
   Includes bibliographical references and index.
   ISBN 0-8247-8496-0 (alk. paper)
   1. Sunscreens (Cosmetics) I. Lowe. N.J. (Nicholas J.)
II. Sunscreens.
   [DNLM: 1. Sunscreening Agents. QV 63 P578]
RS431.S94P49 1991
616.5'061-- --dc20
DNLM / DLC
for Library of Congress   90-14117
                                                CIP

This book is printed on acid-free paper.

MARCEL DEKKER, INC.
270 Madison Avenue, New York, New York 10016

Current printing (last digit):
10 9 8 7 6 5 4 3 2 1

PRINTED IN THE UNITED STATES OF AMERICA

Preface

It has become evident that acute and chronic exposure to sunlight is hazardous to the skin. Much of the damage is induced by ultraviolet wavelengths between 290 and 400 nanometers. The most photoactive and damaging wavelengths lie within the UVB range, between 290 and 320 nanometers. However, more recently it has been determined that UVA wavelengths– 320 to 400 nanometers– may produce significant changes in the skin, particularly when exposed chronically to UVA.

Because of the knowledge that ultraviolet radiation can produce an increased incidence of skin cancer, pigment changes, photoaging, and photosensitivity reactions, the development of sunscreens has become of great importance for the population at large. There is good documentation from both animal and some human studies that the regular use of sunscreens will reduce the damaging effects of ultraviolet radiation on the skin.

Sunscreens were first developed as long ago as 1928. These early sunscreens contained a combination of salicylate and cinnamate. Further developments included the introduction of para-amino benzoic acid (PABA) in 1943 and in the 1950s and 1960s a number of PABA derivatives. Most of these sunscreen chemicals are effective at filtering UVB wavelengths. The subsequent development of UVA sunscreen chemicals includes benzophenones, anthralinates, and, more recently, dibenzoyl methanes. As a result of different combinations of these sunscreens, it is now possible to provide effective protection against UVB and, to a somewhat lesser degree, UVA irradiation.

This book attempts to summarize some of the important aspects of sunscreen evaluation and usage to assist practicing physicians in providing advice for their patients on sun protection.

Nicholas J. Lowe

Contents

Contributors

Teresa D. Bourget Skin Research Foundation of California, Santa Monica, California

Vincent A. DeLeo Department of Dermatology, College of Physicians and Surgeons of Columbia University, New York, New York

Sydney H. Dromgoole Herbert Laboratories, Santa Ana, California

Michele C. Duggan Treatment Skin Care Department, Avon Products, Inc., Suffern, New York

John H. Epstein Department of Dermatology, University of California Medical Center, San Francisco, California

Annette Gottlieb Division of Dermatology, UCLA School of Medicine, Los Angeles, California

Leonard C. Harber Department of Dermatology, College of Physicians and Surgeons of Columbia University, New York, New York

Kays Kaidbey Department of Dermatology, University of Pennsylvania, Philadelphia, Pennsylvania

Albert M. Kligman Department of Dermatology, University of Pennsylvania, Philadelphia, Pennsylvania

Lorraine H. Kligman Department of Dermatology, University of Pennsylvania, Philadelphia, Pennsylvania

Lincoln Krochmal Pharmaceutical Research and Development Division, Bristol-Myers Squibb Company, Buffalo, New York

Nicholas J. Lowe Skin Research Foundation of California, Santa Monica, and Division of Dermatology, UCLA School of Medicine, Los Angeles, California

Howard I. Maibach Department of Dermatology, University of California Medical Center, San Francisco, California

Sergio Nacht Research and Development, Advanced Polymer Systems Inc., Redwood City, California

Mudhukar A. Pathak Harvard Medical School and Department of Dermatology, Massachusetts General Hospital, Boston, Massachusetts

Janet H. Prystowsky Department of Dermatology, College of Physicians and Surgeons of Columbia University, New York, New York

Stewart B. Siskin Pharmaceutical Research and Development Division, Bristol-Myers Squibb Company, Buffalo, New York

Joseph W. Stanfield Pharmaceutical Research and Development Division, Bristol-Myers Squibb Company, Buffalo, New York

Robert S. Stern Harvard Medical School and Department of Dermatology, Beth Israel Hospital, Boston, Massachusetts

James M. Wilmott* Skin Care, Avon Products, Inc., Suffern, New York

Antony R. Young Institute of Dermatology, United Medical and Dental Schools of Guy's and St. Thomas's Hospitals, University of London, London, England

Alexander P. Znaiden Skin Care, Avon Products, Inc., Suffern, New York

---

*Current affiliation: Hair and Skin Care, Dow Brands, Inc., Minneapolis, Minnesota

Physician's Guide
to Sunscreens

I
INTRODUCTION

1
The Need for Photoprotection

NICHOLAS J. LOWE *Skin Research Foundation of California, Santa Monica, California, and UCLA School of Medicine, Los Angeles, California*

The increasing need for sunscreen protection agents to be used by the general population of the United States has become evident over the last several years. In a population that spends more recreational time in the sun, there is a growing awareness of the harmful effects of sunlight exposure resulting in increasing incidence of skin carcinogenesis, accelerated skin aging, and other cutaneous changes including pigmentation anomalies, precancerous lesions such as actinic keratoses as well as melanoma and nonmelanoma skin cancers.

An effective public education campaign has been undertaken by the American Academy of Dermatology in the United States to inform the public of the hazards of sun exposure, particularly the increased risk of skin cancer resulting from severe sunburn reactions. This problem is reduced by sunscreen use.

The hazards of severe sunburns in childhood resulting in an increasing incidence of malignant melanoma have highlighted the importance of effective sunscreen protection from an early stage of childhood.

I. THE NEED FOR PHOTOPROTECTION

A. Photoaging

Repetitive sun exposure can result in skin changes known as photoaged skin. The clinical changes that are seen in photoaged skin differ from those of normally aged skin in some protected sites. There is increased wrinkling, elastosis, solar comedones, pigmentary changes, and precancerous and cancerous skin lesions.

B. Ultraviolet (UV) Wavelengths

In addition to the harmful effects of UVB wavelengths (290–320 nm), there is growing evidence of the harmful effects of UVA (320–400 nm). UVB has been shown to be the most significant causal factor for the formation of skin cancers and a significant component of skin aging. Interesting studies in mouse models suggest that UVB may be responsible for a fine wrinkling of the skin, whereas UVA is capable of causing skin sagging. Whether this has relevance for human skin remains to be determined.

There is evidence that UVA by itself will produce skin damage in human skin including release of vascular mediators, a change in Langerhan's cell population. In susceptible patients, photosensitizing skin diseases as well as photosensitivity reactions occur from certain drugs and chemicals.

Subsequent chapters detail the different sunscreening chemicals that have been developed to absorb both UVB and UVA wavelengths. Combinations of these sunscreens continue to be refined to give broad-spectrum protection against both UVB and UVA wavelengths.

C. Other Environmental Factors and Ultraviolet

In addition to the current awareness of the current dangers of sun exposure, concern is presently being expressed about the increasing depletion of the stratospheric ozone layer. This may result in future increased ultraviolet radiation penetration of the earth's atmosphere. Shorter (UVC) wavelengths of ultraviolet will also increase as a result of ozone depletion.

It is predicted that there will be significant increased incidence of skin carcinogenesis should further ozone layer depletion occur.

D. Infrared Wavelengths

In addition to the risks of increasing ultraviolet from ozone depletion, another area of potential importance, as regards increasing skin carcinogenic risk as well as increasing accelerated skin aging, is infrared radiation to the skin.

Experiments show that infrared radiation in animals can increase ultraviolet-induced skin carcinogenesis as well as produce direct skin-aging changes. The currently effective protection against infrared radiation include the use of sunscreens that contain a powder such as titanium dioxide. Such powders reflect the infrared radiation and obviously must be applied in a sufficient layer to allow adequate protection. Some sunscreens now combine conventional UVB and UVA sunscreen chemical filters with titanium dioxide powders in an attempt to provide broad protection against ultraviolet and infrared radiation.

E. Higher SPF Sunscreens

The continued pursuit of outdoor activity by the general population requires the use of sunscreens with sufficient protection factors to protect the individual against a full day's exposure. In the southern parts of the United States, in the summer months, an SPF factor of 30 may be required to protect against a full day's exposure. These higher SPF sunscreens are now readily available.

Refinements of sunscreening chemicals and vehicles continue to be made and the subsequent chapters in this book will review both the formulation of sunscreens as well as their evaluation. In addition, important photobiological aspects relating to the skin will be discussed.

II
PHOTOBIOLOGICAL
ASPECTS

2

Biological Effect of Sunlight

JOHN H. EPSTEIN *University of California Medical Center, San Francisco, California*

I. INTRODUCTION

This volume is concerned with all aspects of sunscreens. The primary purpose for the existence of these agents is to protect human skin against the damaging effects of the sun's rays. This chapter is concerned with these adverse effects.

II. RADIATION

The electromagnetic spectrum emitted by the sun ranges from the very short cosmic rays to the very long radio waves and beyond. The ultraviolet (UV) rays which comprise the shortest of the nonionizing rays are responsible for most of the photocutaneous changes that occur (Table 1). They have been divided into three categories (1). The shortest UVC rays extend from 100 nm to 280 nm. No wavelengths shorter than 290 nm (288 nm) reach the earth's surface from the sun primarily due to filtration by ozone. Thus though UVC is quite photoactive, it does not constitute a risk to the general population. It can be somewhat hazardous in certain occupations such as welding where some UVC is emitted from artificial sources (2). In contrast, some of the mid UV or UVB rays (290–320 nm) penetrate the ozone layer and are responsible for most of the cutaneous photobiological events induced by exposure to the sun (3). These rays inhibit DNA, RNA, and protein synthesis and mitosis formation, labalise lysosomal and cellular membranes, are mutagenic, and induce early and delayed erythema responses. Chronic UVB exposure damages dermal connective tissue and is the primary carcinogenic stimulus for nonmelanoma skin cancers. Though delayed erythema is usually considered a sunburn reaction, all of the

9

Table 1   Nonionizing Radiation

UVC	100–280 (290) nm
UVB	280 (290)–315 (320) nm
UVA	315 (320)–400 nm
Visible	400–800 nm
Infrared	800–1700 nm

acute phototoxic events noted should be included in this concept. Beneficial effects include new pigment formation, which provides some protection and initiation of the vitamin D cascade, which is important to calcium metabolism. The UVB effects are direct in nature and do not require intermediate photosensitizers. These rays do not pass through window glass as a rule. Thus a sturdy piece of window glass will prevent all of these responses.

The long or near UVA rays (320–400 nm) do pass through window glass and produce a significant number of photobiological effects (4). In contrast to UVB, UVA induces its effects indirectly, requiring oxygen (5,6). Actually the UVA spectrum may have to be divided into at least three parts. The shorter rays between 315 or 320 and 327 nm appear to act directly on cell structures like UVB. Between 327 and 347 nm both direct and indirect effects occur, being more direct toward the 327 nm and indirect toward the 347 nm end of the spectrum. At 335 nm, the contribution of each effect is equal. Between 347 and 400 nm the effects are indirect.

UVA rays induce an immediate erythema which diminishes within 2 hours and a delayed erythema response which reaches a peak at 6 hours (7). This is in contrast to the UVB delayed erythema which tends to reach a peak in 12 to 24 hours. These rays also induce an immediate pigment-darkening reaction and new melanin pigment formation. For people who tan well (type IV skin) it requires more energy to induce an erythema than a tan (6). In fair-complexioned people, about the same amount of energy is required for both the erythema and the new pigment formation responses. The UVA tan response is not associated with epidermal hyperplasia and provides much less of a protection effect against a UVB-induced erythema than the UVB-induced tan (6).

The visible rays are used primarily for vision, though they can induce reactions with certain chemical molecules. The infrared rays supply heat and can induce certain skin changes such as cellular damage and erythema ab igne (8–10).

III.   GOTTHUS DRAPER LAW (11)

This is the primary law of photochemistry and photobiology. It states that non-ionizing radiation must be absorbed to induce a photochemical and thus a subsequent photobiological reaction. As a corollary, the radiation-absorbing molecule, chromophore, photosensitizer, etc., must be present at the time of irradiation for a response to occur.

IV. DEFINITIONS (12)

A. Absorption Spectrum

The rays absorbed by a molecule or a combination of molecules with a greater or lesser efficiency constitute the absorption spectrum of that molecule or those combinations of molecules.

B. Action Spectrum

The wavelengths that are absorbed by a molecule that induce a specific photochemical and/or photobiological reaction with greater or lesser efficiency constitute the action spectrum for that specific reaction. As a corollary, the action spectrum must be included in the absorption spectrum of the photosensitizing molecule since the energy must be absorbed to produce any action.

C. Photosensitivity (13)

Photosensitivity is the broad term used for adverse responses to nonionizing radiation. These reactions may be phototoxic or photoallergic in nature.

Phototoxicity

Phototoxicity is common. It will occur in everyone if enough energy, and in the case of photosensitized reactions, enough of the photosensitizing molecules are present. It is general, characterized by an erythema, usually delayed in onset, followed by hyperpigmentation and desquamation. Thus it simulates the ordinary sunburn response. In fact, the sunburn reaction to UVB rays is the most common of all phototoxic responses.

The mechanisms of phototoxicity are somewhat complicated and may take one of several forms. As with UVB reactions they may result from specific damage to macromolecules such as DNA, RNA, proteins, membranes and the like (3). This is also true of photosensitization by certain molecules such as 8-methoxypsoralen (8-MOP) (14). Such injury can occur with or without the presence of oxygen and the generation of free radicals and superoxides.

In other phototoxic events the presence of oxygen is essential and membrane damage may play a most important role. These are photodynamic reactions and are characteristic of photosensitization by porphyrin molecules, though 8-MOP can also induce such reactions (14).

Another mechanism of phototoxicity depends on the formation of toxic photoproducts. These in turn damage the tissues. This occurs at least at times with chemicals such as chlorpromazine (15).

Photoallergy

In contrast, photoallergy is uncommon. Like all allergies it is dependent upon an acquired altered reactivity dependent upon an immediate humoral or a delayed cell-mediated response. Clinically it is characterized by an immediate wheal and flare or a delayed papular to eczematous reaction.

V. CLINICAL REACTIONS (13)

There is an immense catalog of clinical photosensitivity reactions. In an attempt to bring some order to this complex situation I have divided the problems into three large categories: (1) Those reactions due to a loss or lack of protection; (2) problems due to the presence of a photosensitizing molecule, and (3) the catchall of the responses not due to a loss or lack of protection or the presence of a photosensitizer.

A. Loss or Lack of Protection

The primary protection the skin has against the damaging effects of the sun is melanin pigmentation. The primary problems in this category are related to the presence or absence of melanin. Included in this group are the following problems.

1. *Occulocutaneous Albinism (16)*: In this condition the melanocytes are present but there is a complete or partial deficiency in the tyrosinase activity which is responsible for melanin formation.
2. *Vitiligo (16)*: Vitiligo is characterized by a loss of melanocytes. Thus the photosensitivity is due to the lack of cells to provide the pigmentary system.
3. *Phenylketonuria (16,17) and Chidiak Higashi Diseases (18)*: In both of these diseases the photosensitivity is the result of pigment dilution.
4. *Xeroderma Pigmentosum (XP) (19-21)*: These genetically inherited problems are due to enzymatic inabilities to repair ultraviolet (UV) damaged DNA rather than a pigmentary defect.
5. *Type 1 and 2 Skin (22)*: This category also contains the most common of all the photosensitivity conditions that occur in the light-complexioned individual who sunburns readily and with repeated such injury develops chronic sun damage and skin cancers (23-26).
6. *Action Spectrum*: The reactions in this group are phototoxic and the action spectrum is in the UVB range (24-26).

7. *Therapy and Prevention (22)*: Treatment in this category consists of removal of the precancerous and cancerous tumors that occur with the chronic damage. However, prevention can play a much more important role. This should include avoidance of the midday sun between 10 a.m. and 3 p.m. because of the concentration of the UVB rays during that time; the wearing of protective clothing such as hats and tightly woven garments; and the use of the excellent sunscreens and blocks which are discussed elsewhere in this volume.

B. Photosensitized Reactions

The second clinical category consists of photosensitized reactions. The photosensitizer in this context will be considered a molecule which absorbs the sun's or artificially produced nonionizing radiation and as a result of this process induces an adverse response in the skin. The photosensitizer may be endogenous or exogenous in origin.

1. The porphyrins are the only well-established photosensitizers manufactured by the human body. These are pyrrole ring structures that are essential to cellular metabolism throughout the body. Among other things, the heme part of hemoglobin is formed by these molecules. However, in the group of diseases named the porphyrias, large amounts of porphyrins are made in the erythropoietic (bone marrow) and/or the hepatic (liver) tissues (27). In these states, the porphyrins are not associated with iron and are potent photosensitizers. As such, they induce cutaneous changes ranging from marked photodestruction of the skin and underlying tissues to simple hyperpigmentation, depending on sun exposure and the amount of porphyrin molecules available. The cutaneous changes are due to photodynamic phototoxic responses, and the primary action spectrum is found between 400 and 401 nm.

2. Exogenous photosensitizers may get to the skin by topical application (contact) or through the blood stream (systemic).

a. Topical chemicals may cause photosensitivity reactions advertently, as occurs with tars and psoralen compounds in the treatment of psoriasis and vitiligo, or inadvertently, as occurs with the psoralen molecules in plants and perfumes, halogenated salicylanilides in deodorant soaps, sulfonamide and phenothiazine medications, and so on. In addition, contact photosensitizers are found in moisturizing creams, aftershave lotions, and industrial materials such as polycyclic hydrocarbons contacted in the petrochemical industry, the making of tar products, contactants in agriculture and animal husbandry and the like (13,14, 28). The reactions are usually phototoxic, though occasionally they are photoallergic in type. The phototoxic responses are characterized by erythema and edema followed by hyperpigmentation and desquamation.

Photoallergic photocontact reactions are uncommon. As exceptions, the halogenated salicylanilides (29), musk ambrette (30–32) and 6-methylcoumarin

(33,34), produce primarily photoallergic responses (14). These allergic photo-contact reactions are all delayed hypersensitivity responses.

The action spectrum for these reactions, whether they are phototoxic or photoallergic in nature, usually falls in the UVA range between 320 and 400 nm.

b. Systemically administered chemicals also may induce photosensitivity reactions advertently, as occurs with the use of psoralen compounds in the treatment of vitiligo and psoriasis, or inadvertently, which is the usual case (35,36). These inadvertent photoreactions are generally induced by commonly used medications including antibacterial sulfonamides, thiazide diuretics, sulfonylurea antidiabetic drugs, phenothiazines, certain broad-spectrum antibiotics, and the nonsteroidal antiinflammatory drugs (NAIDS). Of the antibiotics essentially all but minocycline are photosensitizers (37). However, doxycycline and demethyl-chloretracycline are by far the most potent photosensitizers (36,37). Benoxy-prophen was a very potent NAIDS photosensitizer (38–40), but it has been removed from the market. A number of the presently available NAIDS are photosensitizers and will induce acute reactions (41,42). Also some of them have induced low-grade photosensitivity reactions resulting in a pseudoporphyria clinical pattern in the skin. The thiazide diuretics are responsible for more photosensitivity reactions than any of the other commonly used drugs, because they are the most commonly used of these potent photosensitizers.

Amiodarone is an uncommonly used drug for cardiac stabilization. Over 50% of patients taking this drug have photosensitivity reactions (43). Also a significant number develop a blue-black discoloration of their skin. Apparently this discoloration is due to phagocytosis of degraded cell membranes bound to lipid-soluble amiodarone (44). Photosensitivity may persist after the drug has been withdrawn because of tissue retention of the drug.

The vast majority of these clinical reactions are phototoxic in nature, though occasionally delayed hypersensitivity responses may occur. The action spectrum for both phototoxic and photoallergic reactions usually includes long wavelength UV radiation (14,28,36,45).

C. Protection: Normal and No Known Photosensitizer

Photoreactions not due to deficient protection or the presence of known photosensitizers comprise a catchall of conditions.

1. Allergic and autoimmune conditions—These include the apparent photoallergic diseases, the solar urticarias (46), the polymorphous light eruptions (47–49), and the autoimmune diseases such as lupus erythematosus (LE) (50,51), dermatomyositis (52), pemphigus and pemphigoid (53).

The action spectrum for the solar urticarias ranges from UVC rays to infrared energy depending on the specific disease process (46). The polymorphous light eruptions usually respond adversely to UVB rays (47). However, there is a subset of patients who react primarily to UVA radiation (48). The action spectrum for LE is primarily in the UVB range (50), though fibroblasts from LE patients are abnormally sensitive to UVA (54). The reactivity of dermatomyositis patients appears to be UVB rays (52), and both pemphigus and pemphigoid are sensitive to UVB radiation (53). In these autoimmune diseases the abnormal reactions appear to follow phototoxic injuries.

2. Pellagra and pellagra-like diseases include a dietary deficiency in nicotinic acid and/or tryptophan, which results in a cellular deficiency of nicotinic acid (55). Similar problems can be induced by competitive activity of certain medications such as isoniazide and metabolic deviation of nicotinic acid precursors as may be caused by functioning carcinoid tumor. Also, certain disorders of amino acid metabolism such as Hartnup disease (56), hydroxykynurenemia (57) and congenital tryptophanuria (58) may have abnormalities leading to deficiencies in nicotinic acid formation or utilization. These conditions are characterized by erythema and desquamation following sun exposure. This is followed by a dusky brownish-red discoloration. In chronic cases the skin is thickened, scaly and may have a dusky magenta color (55). The action spectrum for this apparent phototoxic response has not been clarified.

3. Certain recessive degenerative genodermatoses may have photosensitivity components (59). In addition to xeroderma pigmentosum (XP) which was noted earlier in this discussion, Bloom's syndrome, Cockayne's syndrome, and poikiloderma congenitale (Rothmund-Thomson syndrome) all have photosensitivity problems. The responses appear to be phototoxic in nature, but the action spectrum has not been clarified. Skin fibroblasts from patients with Bloom's syndrome have reduced survival after UVB radiation (60). In addition, cells from Cockayne patients are hypersensitive to UV radiation (61).

4. The miscellaneous group is the "catchall" of this catchall category. This group contains a number of diverse conditions including certain photodermatoses and other conditions which may be aggravated by sun exposure.

a. The photodermatoses include hydroa aestivale et vacciniforme. Patients with this syndrome respond adversely to UVA rays (62, 63). Whether this is a phototoxic response has not been determined. Disseminated actinic porokeratosis (DSAP) appears to be a peculiar phototoxic response to UV radiation (64). However the definition of the action spectrum has not been completely clarified.

b. A number of photoaggravated diseases are included in this group. Darier's disease is adversely affected by UVB rays (65, 66). This appears to be a phototoxic process. Familial benign chronic pemphigus does respond abnormally to radiation throughout the UVB and UVA spectrum (67). This also appears to be a phototoxic response. Recent studies indicate that UVB can activate herpes simplex infections in humans (68). The action spectrum for reactions in photosensitive psoriasis, granuloma annulare, and acne rosacea remains undetermined.

However, it should be noted that acne rosacea is one of the most common photosensitive diseases.

VI. SUMMARY

Adverse reactions to the sun's rays have become commonplace due not only to excessive sunbathing habits, but also due to the increasing number of photosensitizers in our environment. The sun is responsible for a significant amount of human morbidity ranging from acute sunburn reactions to skin cancer formation. Photodamage to cutaneous cellular macromolecules and membranes, and generation and/or release of inflammatory mediators are integral parts of this photoinjury. Endogenous and exogenous photosensitizing molecules in our personal and general environments supply further pathways for damage. In addition there are a number of photodermatoses and "photoaggravatable" diseases that add to the potential morbidity induced by sun exposure. Hopefully sophistication in the realm of photoprotection will add significantly to our preventive medicine armamentarium.

REFERENCES

1. Parrish, J. A. The scope of photomedicine, *The Science of Photomedicine* (J. D. Regan and J. A. Parrish, eds.), Plenum Press, New York, (1982), pp. 3–17.
2. Birmingham, D. J. Occupational dermatoses. *Progr. Dermatol., 3*:1–8 (1968).
3. Epstein, J. H. Photomedicine, *The Science of Photobiology, 2nd Ed.* (K. C. Smith, ed.), CRC Press Inc., Boca Raton, FL (1988).
4. Urbach, F. and Gange, R. W. (eds.), *The Biological Effects of UVA Radiation*, Praeger Publ., New York (1986).
5. Peak, M. J. and Peak, J. G. Molecular photobiology of UVA. *The Biological Effects of UVA Radiation* (F. Urbach and R. W. Gange, eds.), Praeger Publ., New York (1986), pp. 42–56.
6. Gange, R. W., Park, Y.-K., Auletta, M., Kagetsu, N., Blackett, A. D., and Parrish, J. A. Action spectra for cutaneous responses to ultraviolet radiation, *The Biological Effects of UVA Radiation* (F. Urbach and R. W. Gange, eds.), Praeger Publ., New York (1986), pp. 57–67.
7. Whitman, G. B., Leach, E. E., Deleo, V. A., and Harber, L. C. Comparative response to UVA radiation in humans and guinea pigs, *The Biological Effects of UVA Radiation* (F. Urbach and R. W. Gange, eds.), Praeger Publ., New York (1986), pp. 79–86.
8. Cross, F. On a turf (peat) fire cancer. Malignant change sumerpimposed on erythema ab igne. *Proc. Roy. Soc. Med., 60*:1307–1308 (1967).
9. Arrington, J. H. III. Thermal keratoses and squamous carcinoma in situ associated with erythema ab igne. *Arch. Dermatol., 115*:1226–1228 (1979).

10. Kligman, L. H. Intensification of ultraviolet-induced dermal damage by infrared radiation. *Arch. Fur Dermatologische Forschung, 272*:229–238 (1982).
11. Harber, L. C. and Bickers, D. R. *Photosensitivity Diseases, Principles of Diagnosis and Treatment*, W. B. Saunders Co., Philadelphia (1981), pp. 24–25.
12. Epstein, J. H. Photoallergy and photoimmunology, *Dermatologic Immunology and Allergy* (J. Stone, ed.), C. V. Mosby Co., St. Louis, MO (1985), pp. 629–640.
13. Epstein, J. H. Phototoxicity and photoallergy, *Sunlight and Man* (M. A. Pathak et al., eds.), University of Tokyo Press, Tokyo (1974), pp. 459–477.
14. Epstein, J. H. and Wintroub, B. U. Photosensitivity due to drugs. *Drugs, 30*: 42–57 (1985).
15. Kochevar, I. E. Phototoxicity mechanisms: Chlorpromazine photosensitized damage to DNA and cell membranes. *J. Invest. Dermatol.,* 77:59–64 (1981).
16. Bolognia, J. L. and Pawelek, J. M. Biology of hypopigmentation. *J. Am. Acad. Dermatol., 19*:217–255 (1988).
17. Knox, W. E. Phenylketonuria, *Metabolic Basis of Inherited Disease* (J. B. Stanbury, J. B. Wyngaarden, and D. S. Fredrickson, eds.), McGraw-Hill, New York (1972), pp. 266–295.
18. Windhorst, D. B., Zelickson, A. S., and Good, R. A. A human pigmentary dilution based on a heritable subcellular structural defect—The Chediak-Higashi syndrome. *J. Invest. Dermatol., 50*:9–18 (1968).
19. Cleaver, J. E. Defective repair replication of DNA in xeroderma pigmentosum. *Nature, 218*:652–653 (1968).
20. Epstein, J. H., Fukuyama, K., Reed, W. B., and Epstein, W. L. Defect in DNA synthesis in skin of patients with xeroderma pigmentosum demonstrated in vivo. *Science, 168*:1477–1478 (1970).
21. Kraemer, K. A., Lee, M. M., Scotto, J. Xeroderma pigmentosum: Cutaneous, ocular and neurologic abnormalities in 830 published cases. *Arch. Dermatol., 123*:241–250 (1987).
22. Pathak, M. A., Fitzpatrick, T. B., and Parrish, J. A. Topical and systemic approaches to protection of human skin against harmful effects of solar radiation, *The Science of Photomedicine* (J. D. Regan and J. A. Parrish, eds.), Plenum Press, New York (1982), pp. 441–473.
23. Scotto, J., Fears, T. R., and Fraumeni, J. F. Jr. Incidence of nonmelanoma skin cancer in the United States. U.S. Department of Health, Education and Welfare, Publication Number (NIH) 82-2433 (1981).
24. Urbach, F. Photocarcinogenesis, *The Science of Photomedicine* (J. D. Regan and J. A. Parrish, eds.), Plenum Press, New York (1982), pp. 261–292.
25. Epstein, J. H. Photocarcinogenesis, skin cancer and aging. *J. Am. Acad. Dermatol., 9*:487–502 (1983).
26. Van der Leun, J. UV Carcinogenesis. *Photochem. Photobiol., 39*:861–868 (1984).

27. Poh-Fitzpatrick, M. B. Porphyrias, *Photomedicine, Vol. 1* (E. Ben-Hur and I. Rosenthal, eds.), CRC Press Inc., Boca Raton, FL (1987), pp. 163–178.
28. Harber, L. C., Kochevar, I. E., and Shalita, A. R. Mechanisms of photosensitization to drugs in humans, *The Science of Photomedicine* (J. D. Regan and J. A. Parrish, eds.), Plenum Press, New York (1982), pp. 323–347.
29. Herman, P. S. and Sams, W. M. Jr. *Soap Photodermatitis*, Charles C Thomas, Springfield, IL (1972).
30. Raug, G. J., Storrs, F. J., and Larsen, W. G. Photoallergic contact dermatitis to mens perfume. *Contact Dermatitis, 5*:251–260 (1979).
31. Riovinazzo, V. J., Ichikawa, H., Kochevar, I. E., Armstrong, R. B., and Harber, L. C. Photoallergic contact dermatitis to musk ambrette: Action spectrum in guinea pigs and man. *Photochem. Photobiol., 33*:773–777 (1981).
32. Galosi, A. and Plewig, G. Photoallergic eczema caused by musk ambrette. *Hautarzt, 33*:589–594 (1982).
33. Kaidbey, K. H. and Kligman, A. M. Contact photoallergy to 6-methyl-coumarin in proprietary sunscreens. *Arch. Dermatol., 114*:1709–1710 (1978).
34. Jackson, R. T., Nesbit, L. T., and DeLeo, V. A. 6-Methylcoumarin photo-contact dermatitis. *J. Am. Acad. Dermatol., 2*:124–127 (1980).
35. Epstein, J. H. Chemical phototoxicity in humans. *J. Natl. Cancer Inst., 69*: 265–268 (1982).
36. Toback, A. C. and Anders, J. E. Phototoxicity from systemic agents, *Dermatologic Clinics; Photosensitivity Diseases* (V. A. De Leo, ed.), W. B. Saunders Co., Philadelphia (1986), pp. 223–230.
37. Bjellerup, M., Kjellstrom, T., and Ljunggren, B. Influence of tetracycline phototoxicity on growth of cultured human fibroblasts. *J. Invest. Dermatol., 85*:573–574 (1985).
38. Ferguson, J., Addo, H. A., McGill, P. E. et al. A study of benoxaprofen-induced photosensitivity. *Br. J. Dermatol., 107*:429–442 (1982).
39. Halsey, J. Benoxaprofen side-effect profile in 300 patients. *Br. Med. J., 284*:1365 (1982).
40. Kochevar, I. E., Hoover, K. W., and Gawienowski, M. Benoxaprofen photosensitization of cell membrane disruption. *J. Invest. Dermatol., 82*:214–218 (1984).
41. Diffey, B. L., Daymond, T. J., and Fairgreaves, H. Phototoxic reactions to prixoicam, naproxen, and tiaprofenic acid. *Br. J. Rheumatol., 22*:239–242 (1983).
42. Stern, R. S. and Bigby, M. An expanded profile of cutaneous reactions to nonsteroidal anti-inflammatory drugs. Reports to a specialty-based system for spontaneous reporting of adverse reactions to drugs. *JAMA, 252*:1433–1437 (1984).
43. Diffey, B. L., Chalmers, R. J. G., and Muston, N. L. Photobiology of amiodarone: Preliminary in vitro and in vivo studies. *Clin. Exp. Dermatol., 9*: 248–255 (1984).

44. Zachary, C. B., Slater, D. N., Holt, D. W., Storey, G. C. A., and MacDonald, D. M. The pathogenesis of amiodarone-induced pigmentation and photosensitivity. *Br. J. Dermatol., 110*:451–456 (1984).

45. Elmets, C. Drug induced photoallergy, *Dermatologic Clinics; Photosensitivity Diseases* (V. A. DeLeo, ed.), W. B. Saunders Co., Philadelphia (1986), pp. 231–241.

46. Armstrong, R. B. Solar urticaria, *Dermatologic Clinics; Photosensitivity Diseases* (V. A. DeLeo, ed.), W. B. Saunders Co., Philadelphia (1986), pp. 253–259.

47. Epstein, J. H. Polymorphous light eruption. *J. Am. Acad. Dermatol., 3*: 329–343 (1980).

48. Holzle, E., Plewig, G., Hofmann, C. et al. Polymorphous light eruption: Experimental reproduction of lesions. *J. Am. Acad. Dermatol., 7*:111–125 (1982).

49. Epstein, J. H. Polymorphous light eruption, *Dermatologic Clinics; Photosensitivity Diseases* (V. A. DeLeo, ed.), W. B. Saunders Co., Philadelphia (1986), pp. 243–251.

50. Tuffanelli, D. L. and Epstein, J. H. Chronic cutaneous (discoid) lupus erythematosus, *Dubois' Lupus Erythematosus,* Third Edition (D. J. Wallace, E. L. Dubois, eds.), Lea & Febiger, Philadelphia (1987), pp. 283–301.

51. Hymes, S. R., Jordan, R. E., and Arnett, F. C. Lupus erythematous, *Dermatologic Clinics; Photosensitivity Diseases* (V. A. DeLeo, ed.), W. B. Saunders Co., Philadelphia (1986), pp. 267–276.

52. Caro, I. A dermatologist's view of dermatomyositis. *Clinics in Dermatology; Polymyositis/Dermatomyositis,* Vol. 2, No. 6, (R. D. Sontheimer, ed.), J. D. Lippincott, Philadelphia (1988), pp. 9–14.

53. Cram, D. L. and Kukuyama, K. The immunochemistry of ultraviolet-induced pemphigus and pemphigoid lesions. *Arch. Dermatol., 106*:819–824 (1972).

54. Zamansky, G. B., Minka, D. F., Deal, C. L. et al. The in vitro photosensitivity of lupus erythematosus skin fibroblasts. *J. Immunol., 134*:1571–1576 (1985).

55. Stratigos, J. D. and Katsambas, A. Pellagra: A still existing disease. *Br. J. Dermatol., 96*:99–106 (1977).

56. Baron, D. N., Dent, C. E., Harris, H., Hartz, H., Hart, E. W., and Hepson, J. B. Hereditary pellagra-like skin rash with temporary cerebellar ataxia, constant renal aminoaciduria and other bizarre chemical features. *Lancet, 2*:421–428 (1956).

57. Kromrower, G. M. and Westall, R. Hydroxykinureninuria. *Am. J. Dis. Child., 113*:77–80 (1967).

58. Tada, K., Ito, H., Wada, Y., and Arakawa, T. Congenital tryptophanuria with dwarfism: Toboku. *J. Exp. Med., 80*:118–134 (1963).

59. Bligard, G. A. and Storer, J. S. Photosensitivity in infants and children, *Dermatologic Clinics; Photosensitivity Disease* (V. A. DeLeo, ed.), W. B. Saunders, Co., Philadelphia (1986), pp. 311–320.

60. Zbinden, I. and Cerutti, P. Near ultraviolet sensitivity of skin fibroblasts

of patients with Bloom's syndrome. *Biophys. Res. Commun., 98*:579–587 (1981).

61. Lehmann, A. R., Francis, A. J., and Giannelli, F. Prenatal diagnosis of Cockayne's syndrome. *Lancet, 1*:486–488 (1985).

62. Goldgeier, M. H., Nordland, J. J., and Lucky, A. W. Reproduction of hydroa vacciniforme with UVA. *J. Am. Acad. Dermatol., 9*:278–280 (1983).

63. Halasz, L. L. G., Leach, E. E., Walther, R. R., et al. Hydroa vacciniforme: Induction of lesions with ultraviolet A. *J. Am. Acad. Dermatol., 8*:171–176 (1983).

64. Chernosky, M. E. and Anderson, D. E. Disseminated superficial actinic porokeratosis. *Arch. Dermatol., 99*:401–407 (1969).

65. Shelley, W. B., Arthur, R. P., and Pillsbury, D. M. A view of keratosis follicularis (Darier's disease) as a neoplastic process. *Arch. Dermatol., 80*:332–338 (1959).

66. Penrod, J. M., Everett, M. A., and McCreight, W. G. Observations on keratosis follicularis. *Arch. Dermatol., 82*:367–370 (1960).

67. Cram, D. L., Muller, S. A., and Winkelmann, R. K. Ultraviolet-induced acantholysis in familial benign pemphigus. *Arch. Dermatol., 96*:636–641 (1967).

68. Perna, J. J., Mannix, M. L., Rooney, J. F., Notkins, A. L., and Straus, S. E. Reactivation of latent herpes simplex virus infection by ultraviolet light: A human model. *J. Am. Acad. Dermatol., 17*:473–478 (1987).

3
Ultraviolet Radiation-Induced Skin Aging

LORRAINE H. KLIGMAN and ALBERT M. KLIGMAN *University of Pennsylvania, Philadelphia, Pennsylvania*

I. INTRODUCTION

Recognition of the environmental influences on the aging of human skin has followed a cyclical and often deviant path. In recent years, renewed emphasis has been placed upon the major role of solar ultraviolet radiation in what we now call photoaging. Although a new term, photoaging is not a new concept. Dermatologists of the late 19th century, notably Unna (1) and Dubreuilh (2) described the devastating effects of sunlight on the skin of farmers and sailors compared with the appearance of indoor workers. Appreciation of these findings were gradually lost as the pursuit of deeply tanned skin as an indication of health and well-being developed in western caucasoid cultures. For many years the consequences of overexposure to sunlight were ignored and misnamed. Because serious sunworshippers can look old, even at age 50, with wrinkled, leathery skin, it became customary to regard the worn facial appearance as "premature" aging. The changes were considered merely an acceleration of the natural or intrinsic aging process, differing only quantitatively (3). In contrast, some descriptions of intrinsically aged skin failed to account for the effects of solar radiation on exposed areas of the body (4). To compound the difficulties, biopsies of aged skin were often from very old persons with unknown amounts of sun exposure. The result was a blurred distinction between the characteristics of intrinsic aging and photoaging.

Recent experimental work has concentrated on clarifying past misconceptions. In addition, once again, clinical observations are reconfirming that octogenarians who have avoided sun exposure can still have smooth, unblemished skin, showing only a laxness and deepening of expression lines. On the other hand, photoaged skin displays a variety of neoplasms, deep furrows, extensive sagging with a yellowed, nodular surface marked by telangiectatic traceries. These drastic, visible aspects reflect profound structural dermal alterations that are quite different from those found in protected, intrinsically aged skin (5).

II. PHOTOAGING VERSUS INTRINSIC AGING

A. The Dermal Matrix

Although clinical evidence for photodamage can remain inapparent for many years, ultraviolet-induced changes in elastic fibers can be detected, histologically, as early as the second decade (6). It begins as a marked hyperplasia of relatively normal fibers, leading to accumulations of massive quantities of thickened,

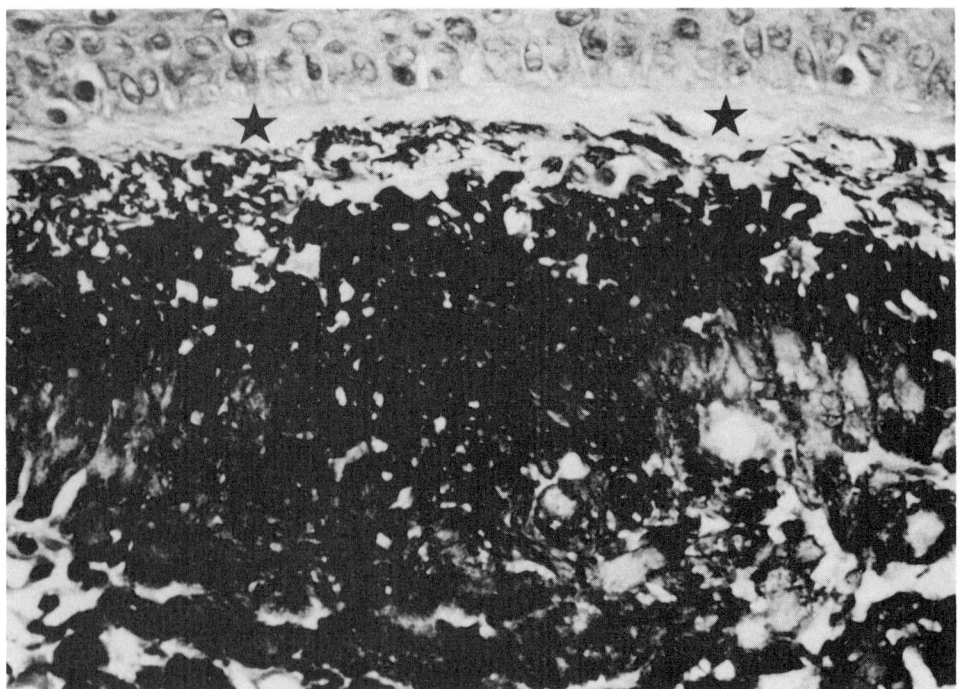

Figure 1 Advanced elastosis in human skin. Amorphous masses of degraded elastic fibers replace most of the collagen. Only a narrow Grenz zone remains (★). Luna's stain (X125).

tangled, degraded fibers which eventually degenerate into an amorphous mass (Fig. 1). Ultrastructurally, the homogeneous elastin matrix begins to appear granular and develops numerous electron lucent areas which impart a motheaten appearance (7). As the photoaging process continues, the matrix disappears, leaving only tangled microfilaments. Elastosis to this degree never occurs in the protected skin of older persons. Instead, intrinsically aged skin shows a modest increase in the number and thickness of elastic fibers (Fig. 2a) and some loss of the fine vertical fibers that, in young skin (Fig. 2b), insert into the basement membrane (3,8). Ultrastructurally, there is deterioration characterized by the development of lacunae which cause a loosening of the aggregated components of mature fibers (7).

Collagen, the major component of dermal connective tissue, also undergoes UV-induced changes. In the past, few collagen-specific histochemical observations were made. Brief descriptions exist which note changes in staining characteristics (9) with emphasis on "basophilic degeneration" of collagen. This has proved to be a misnomer. The bluish stained material in hematoxylin and eosin sections is now recognized as elastosis (10). A late change in photoaging is a substantial loss of collagen as it is replaced by the masses of elastosis (Fig. 1).

Because few systematic studies have been done with humans, the early effects of UV radiation must be inferred from animal experiments. Initially the dermis thickens, as fibroblasts are stimulated to synthesize collagen. With further UV exposure there is a progressive loss of stain in deep bands across the dermis (11). Although there is no consensus on whether UV radiation has a direct effect on collagen (12,13) there is an abundance of experimental evidence suggesting that the UV-induced inflammatory infiltrate is responsible for collagen degradation (12,14-16).

Early biochemical analysis of sun-damaged human skin showed a decrease in insoluble (mature) collagen and an increase in soluble (new) collagen (17). Recent biochemical studies of UV-irradiated human skin suggest these changes may be due to a progressive increase in the ratio of type III to type I collagen (18). In intrinsic aging, however, collagen apparently becomes more highly cross-linked with greater resistance to enzymatic degradation (19,20). Bundle deposition also becomes more dense (21).

The third component of the dermal matrix, the ground substance, is composed of the proteoglycans (PGs) dermatan sulfate and heparan sulfate and the glycosaminoglycan (GAG) hyaluronic acid. Abundant in fetal skin, these decrease rapidly in early life. In protected skin, they remain low throughout most of adult life (17). In photoaged skin, ground substance drastically increases to levels almost matching that of fetal skin (17,22). Other molecules such as fibronectin increase in photoaged skin and bind to the elastotic masses (10).

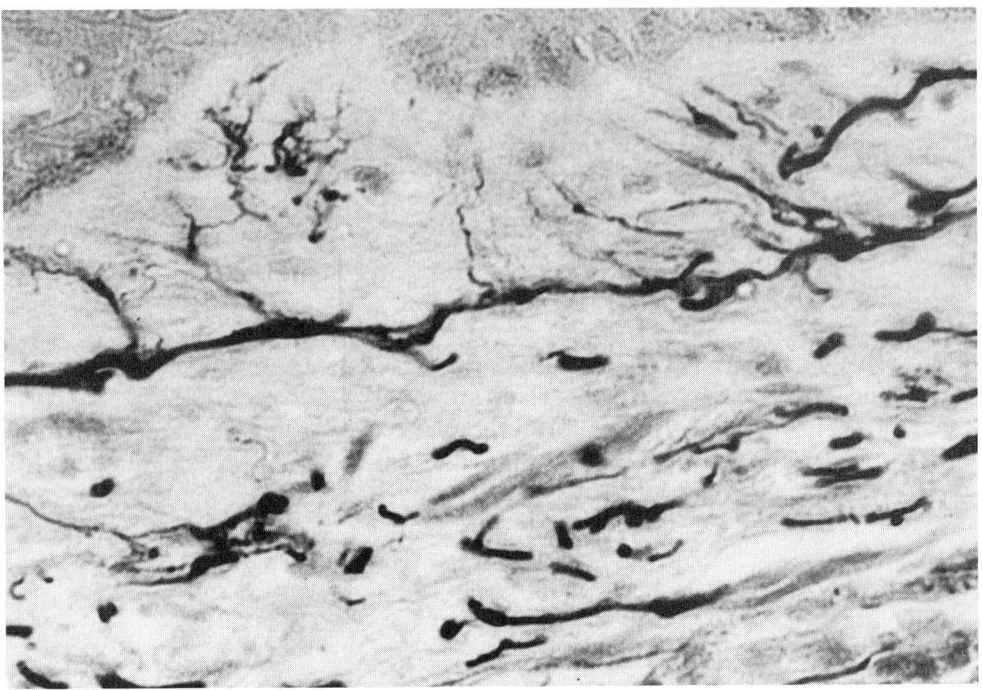

(a)

Figure 2   (a) Protected aged skin with slightly thickened elastic fibers and extensive loss of the vertical fibers that normally insert into the dermal-epidermal
junction. Note the flattened junctional area and lack of rete ridges. Luna's stain
(X380). (b) Young protected skin replete with fine candelabra-like vertical fibers
Orcein (X380).

B. Other Dermal Components

Fibroblasts, especially those of the upper dermis, in chronically sun-exposed skin
are numerous and appear to be in a state of high metabolic activity, as judged by
hypertrophy of the endoplasmic reticulum. The opposite occurs in intrinsic
aging. There are fewer fibroblasts and these are atrophic. Dermal thinning is
characteristic of intrinsic aging whereas the opposite occurs in chronically irradiated skin, at least until endstage photodegradation occurs. In photodamaged
skin, there is also a perivenular histiocytic-lymphocytic infiltrate in which
numerous mast cells, often partially degranulated, are seen in close proximity to
fibroblasts (15). In this chronic "heliodermatitis" (Fig. 3), it is likely that mast
cell-produced mediators, in conjunction with proteolytic enzymes released by

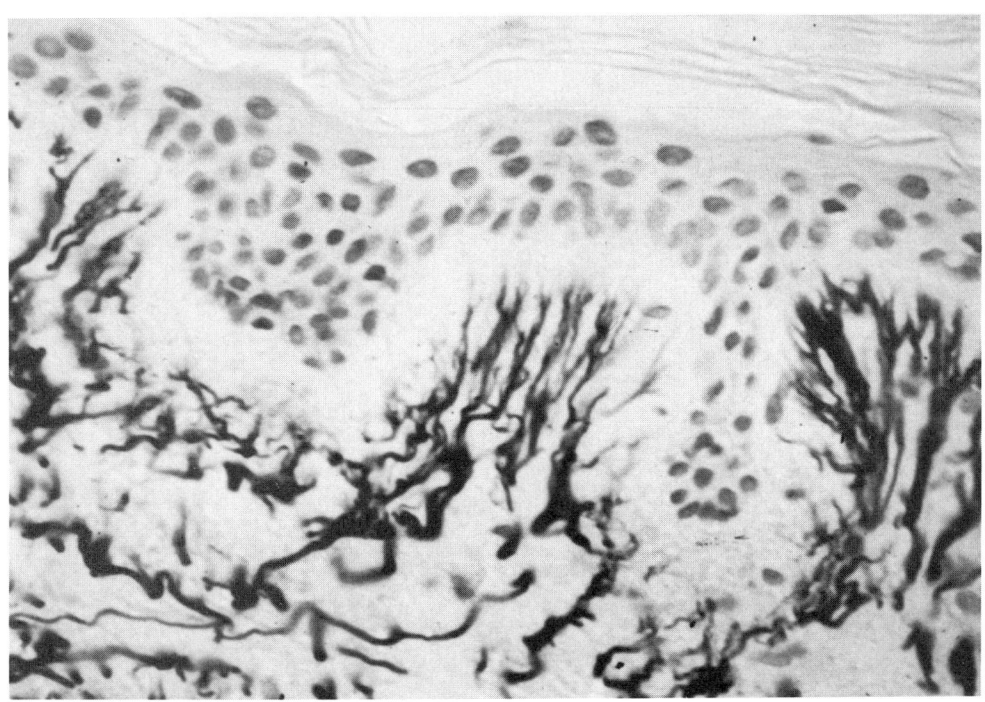

(b)

the infiltrating cells may lead to the degradation of elastic and collagen fibers. In contrast, in chronologic aging, hypocellularity is the rule (23).

The microcirculation with its delicate capillary loops (Fig. 4a) also suffers from sun exposure. Vessels become dilated and tortuous (Fig. 4b), seen on the surface as telangiectases. Finally, they become sparse, with massive loss of the capillary loops and disruption of the horizontal plexus (24). Ultrastructurally, walls of the vessels are greatly thickened by deposition of reduplicated basement membrane-like material, which also contains reticulin fibers (25). In protected aged skin, there is some loss of the subepidermal capillary loops, probably secondary to flattening of the dermal–epidermal junction. The vessels however, are not dilated and the horizontal plexus is largely undisturbed (24,26). Moderate thickening of the vessel walls is occasionally seen in intrinsic aging but in some very old persons, the vessels often have abnormally thin walls (25).

Finally, benign, malignant, and premalignant lesions flourish in photoaged skin. Seborrheic and actinic keratoses, solar lentigos, keratoacanthomas, basal cell epitheliomas and squamous cell carcinomas develop almost exclusively in sun-exposed areas (27). Senile or cherry angiomas are about the only growths that regularly appear in protected aged skin.

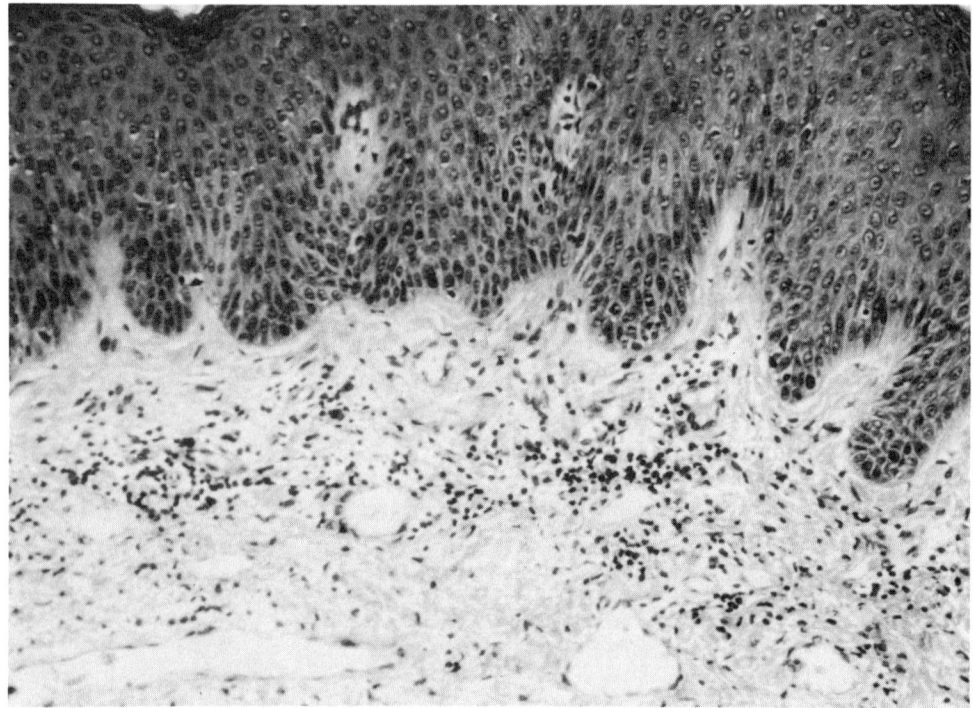

Figure 3 Heliodermatitis in chronically irradiated skin. Note the marked epidermal hyperplasia and severe cellular inflammatory infiltrate. H & E (X380).

In summary, contrary to the usual textbook statement that sun-damaged skin is thin and atrophic, ongoing photoaging is characterized by "more" not "less" until end-stage photodamage in the very elderly. Hypertrophy rules in photoaging: epidermis thickens and sprouts neoplasms, sebaceous glands enlarge (4, 28), elastic fibers multiply, collagen synthesis is stimulated, ground substance increases while inflammatory cells abound and vessel walls thicken.

II. EXPERIMENTAL STUDIES

Photoaging in humans is a slowly evolving process, taking decades to become clinically apparent and many more years to develop all of the manifestations, whether microscopically or biochemically. Furthermore, the UV dosimetry of human sun exposure is impossible to quantify with any degree of accuracy. Systematic studies require animal models for practical as well as ethical reasons. The hairless mouse has proved to be a relevant model for human photoaging. The

UV-induced changes, ranging from acute responses (29) to those associated with chronic exposure such as tumorigenesis (30) and connective tissue damage (31, 32) are comparable to those in human skin.

A. UVB and Photoaging

UVB (280–320 nm) is well known to be responsible for erythema, DNA damage, and skin cancer. Some evidence was provided by Sams et al. (33) that it was also effective in damaging connective tissue. These authors produced a modest amount of elastic fiber hyperplasia in haired mice after a severely damaging dose of 30 to 50 minimal erythema doses. Although their UV source emitted some UVC (200–280 nm), it was assumed that the effective waveband was the longer wavelength UVB which is capable of penetrating into the dermis. With the hairless mouse it has been possible to produce extensive connective tissue photodamage with far lower doses. A bank of FS Westinghouse "sunlamps" is a convenient high-energy source of predominantly UVB radiation. The quantity of UVA emitted is inconsequential with regard to connective tissue damage (14). The small UVC component can be filtered out effectively with a cellulose triacetate film. Normally, the hairless mouse has very little elastic tissue. Nevertheless, it was possible to produce severe elastosis (Fig. 5) with a total of 5 J/cm^2 delivered as 2 minimal erythema doses (MED) per exposure, thrice weekly for approximately 30 weeks (14). Ultrastructural changes (Fig. 6) in the elastic fibers bore a remarkable similarity to those seen in photodamaged human skin (34). In irradiated animals, fibroblasts became more numerous. Ultrastructurally, they appeared to be metabolically active, producing increased quantities of collagen that contributed to a thickening of the dermis. Reticulin fibers, normally limited to the basement membrane zones, were prominent throughout the upper dermis, an indication of new collagen synthesis (31). A decreased affinity for van Gieson's stain suggested severe damage to mature collagen. The histologic findings were confirmed by electron microscopy. In addition to a fraying and partial dissolution of large collagen fibers, there were numerous fibers of small diameters that may be newly synthesized collagen. Recently, UVB-irradiated hairless mouse skin has been examined with biochemical techniques. In one study, using cyanogen bromide digestion of whole skin, an early and progressive increase in the ratio of type III to total collagen was reported (35). It was implied that this was due to an increase in type III collagen. Another study (Kligman L.H., Gebre M., Alper R., Kefalides N.A.: *J. Invest. Dermatol.* 93:210–214, 1989) using pepsin digestion of isolated collagen, showed a progressive increase in total collagen during chronic irradiation but with a return to control levels after months of irradiation. There was no increase in the ratio of type III to total collagen until the loss of total collagen was detected. Schwarz et al. (36) have also reported no change in the ratio in UVB-irradiated mouse

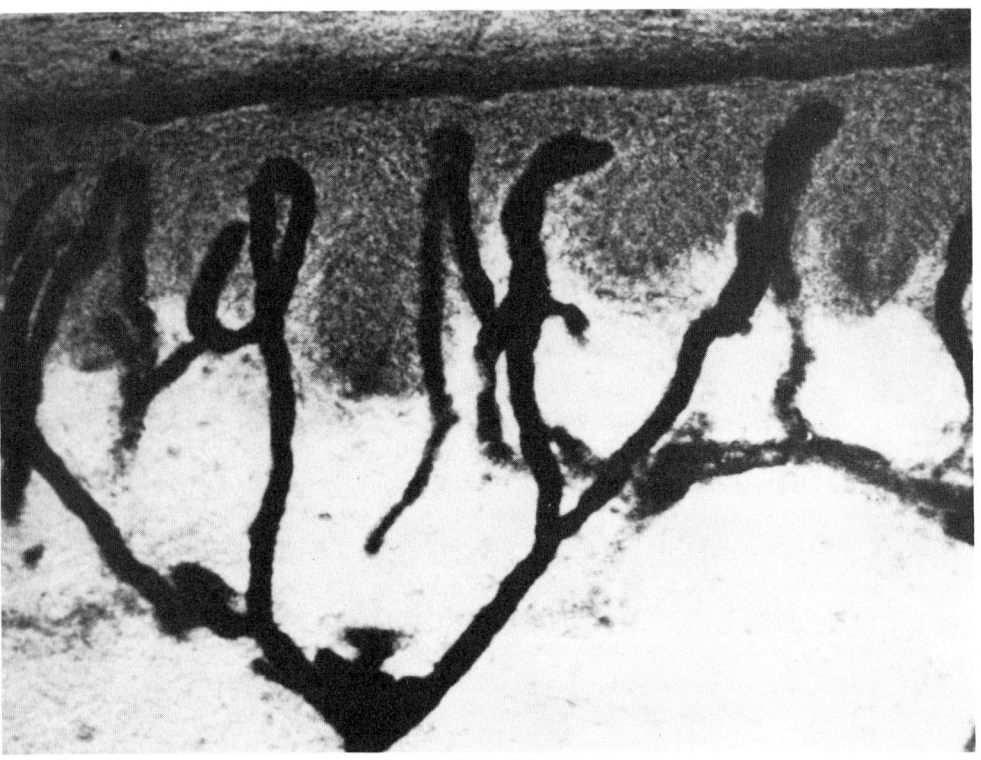

(a)

Figure 4   Superficial vasculature. (a) Protected young adult skin with well-defined capillary loops. (b) Dilated vessels with disrupted architecture in photo-damaged skin. Alkaline phosphatase stain (X100).

skin. These results suggest that both types I and III collagen increase proportionally until the end-stage of photodamage when there is loss of type I collagen.

A compilation of histochemical and biochemical damage suggests that photodamage to the collagen matrix is at least biphasic. Early on, fibroblasts are stimulated to produce more collagen, with the new soluble collagen, whether type I or type III, having little affinity for van Gieson's stain, but appearing as "reticulin" fibers. After long-term chronic irradiation when mature collagen is lost at a faster rate than fibroblasts can replace it, the dermis thins, becoming atrophic in end-stage photoaging.

The third component of the mouse dermis, the GAGs and PGs of the ground substance, as in humans, become greatly increased with chronic UV radiation.

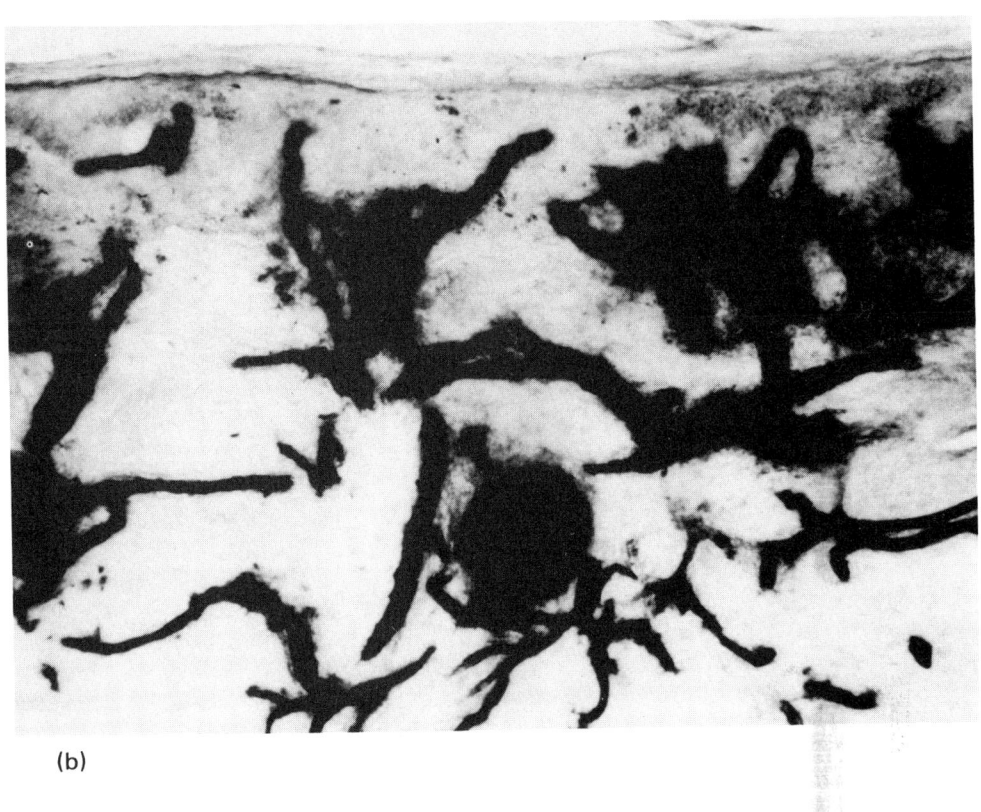

(b)

B. UVA and Photoaging

Recently, it has been shown that acute exposure to UVA (320–400 nm) can, like UVB, produce erythema (37) and damage blood vessels (38). Because such effects require doses that may be 1000 times greater than UVB, the role of UVA in photoaging was thought to be negligible. However, UVA is present in sunlight in amounts that can be 100 to 500 times that of UVB. Furthermore, its longer wavelengths allow more of it to reach the dermis than does UVB. These considerations make it important to examine the effects of UVA alone in comparison with UVB (14). Hairless mice were irradiated with a solar simulator filtered to provide UVA with a spectral distribution similar to that of solar UVA. Animals irradiated with this source for 34 weeks, with a total UVA dose of 3000 J/cm^2 developed a significant degree of elastosis. Although the deposition of elastic fibers was less dense than that produced by a total UVB dose of 5 J/cm^2, the elastosis extended more deeply into the dermis (Fig. 7). UVA from a black

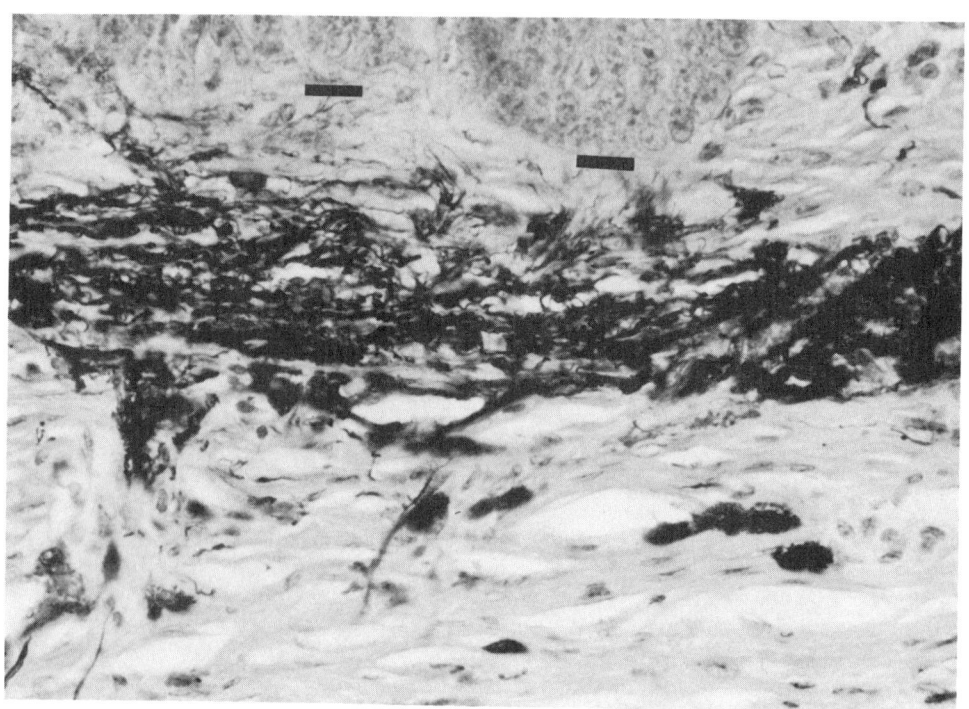

Figure 5 Mouse skin. Elastosis induced by chronic exposure to UVB. Luna's stain (×380). Dermal–epidermal junction = (–).

light source (340–400 nm), with peak emission at approximately 365 nm, produced only mild elastic fiber hyperplasia despite a total UVA dose of 13,000 J/cm^2. This strongly suggests that the UVA wavelengths of 320–340 nm, abundant in solar UVA but lacking in the black light spectrum, are those most responsible for UVA-induced photodamage. However, the longer wavelengths of solar-simulating UVA (>340 nm) cannot be ignored. Recent studies have shown elastic fiber hyperplasia and increased GAGs with high, but not unrealistic doses (39). In contrast to UVB, solar-simulating UVA had little or no histologic effect on collagen. Supporting the hypothesis that it is the proteolytic enzymes of the inflammatory infiltrate that degrade collagen, UVA did not induce inflammation.

   Like UVB, UVA radiation produced an increase in GAGs and PGs as visualized with Mowry's stain. The distribution, however, was different. Whereas UVB produced granular blue staining material localized in the upper dermis, UVA-induced GAGs and PGs were deposited throughout, imparting a bluish hue to

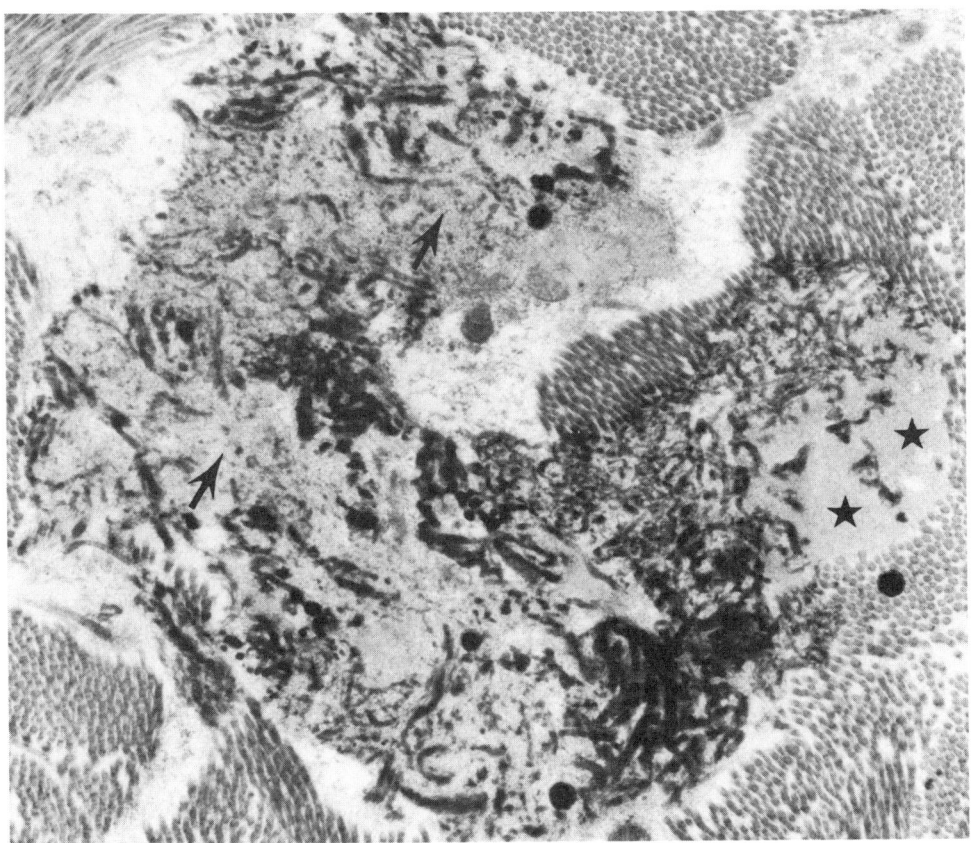

Figure 6 Elastotic clump of fibers in mouse skin irradiated for 30 weeks. Most of the electron dense matrix is degraded, leaving granular (→) and amorphous (★) residues. Glutaraldehyde-osmium-tannic acid staining.

the entire dermis. Additionally, densely staining material was deposited at the dermal-epidermal junction.

These findings provided compelling evidence that UVA radiation, especially solar-simulating UVA, is capable of inducing profound photodamage to dermal connective tissue. Furthermore, the dose used in these experiments was realistic in terms of human exposure. For example, a 1-hour exposure at midday in June at 40 degrees north latitude will provide approximately 10 J/cm^2 UVA. Within 4 years, summertime exposure alone could result in the accumulation of 3000 J/cm^2. Of concern also is the greatly increased absorption of UVA by persons

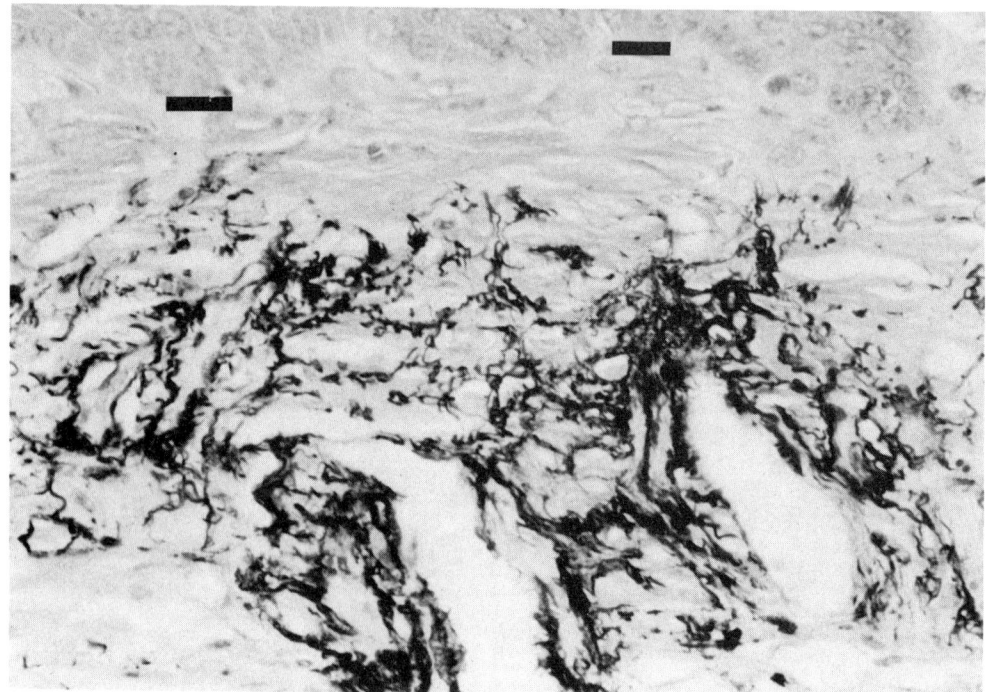

Figure 7 Mouse skin. Delicate, deeply deposited UVA-induced elastosis. Luna's stain (X380). Dermal--epidermal junction = (–).

protected with a sunscreen that filters out only UVB. Many more hours in the sun are now possible without the warning of a sunburn.

C. Solar-Simulating Radiation and Photoaging

Although the effects of UVA alone are interesting from a scientific point of view, it is the cumulative effect of the entire ultraviolet spectrum that is of prime concern. In the study described above, a group of animals was exposed to full-spectrum solar-simulating radiation (14). The total UVB dose, delivered during the 34-week experiment, was approximately 5 J/cm^2 with a 100-fold more solar-simulating UVA. In some aspects, the photodamage reflected the influence of both wavebands, whereas in others, it was like UVB alone. Elastosis was severe but not confined to the upper dermis as with UVB. More dense than UVA elastosis, it extended deeply into the dermis. Collagen was damaged to an extent comparable to UVB alone. GAGs were equal to or slightly increased compared with UVB-irradiated tissue, with darkly stained material at the dermal-epidermal junction, providing evidence for the additional effect of UVA.

D. Prevention of Photoaging: Sunscreens

In the hairless mouse model, broad-spectrum sunscreens, with a sun protection factor (SPF) of 15, provided effective protection against ultraviolet-induced connective tissue damage. This was especially true for animals irradiated with UVB at approximately 6 MED (minimal erythema dose) per exposure (31). Histologic specimens were virtually indistinguishable from normal age-matched controls. Animals irradiated with solar-simulating radiation (~2 MED UVB + UVA) and protected by the same sunscreens showed some mild dermal damage (14). Elastosis was prevented, but elastic fibers were mildly hyperplastic. Collagen appeared undamaged, and although dermal cellularity was increased, massive inflammation did not occur. GAGs were slightly but not remarkably increased compared with unirradiated controls.

In both experiments, the sunscreen applications began at the time of the first exposure. This does not conform to human practice where sunscreens are generally not used until some degree of photodamage (such as the first wrinkle or actinic keratosis) is clinically visible. By that time, the connective tissue has already sustained severe photodamage. Previously, it was believed that this damage was irreversible. Early studies with hairless mice demonstrated that considerable repair could occur within a few months, even after extensive photodamage, if the UV exposures were stopped (31). Broad regions of new collagen were deposited in the subepidermal dermis, pushing downward the old elastotic material (Fig. 8a). The new collagen was normal, histochemically and ultrastructurally; new elastic fibers in this region were sparse and delicate as in unirradiated tissue. Interestingly, evidence for similar repair is seen in human skin when former sunworshippers avoid further sun exposure (Fig. 8b).

Because of these findings, it was of interest to determine if the skin could repair itself in a like manner under conditions that simulated human experience (11). Groups of animals were irradiated for a total of 30 weeks with UVB (3 MED per exposure). Sunscreens of SPF 6 and 15 were applied to separate groups after 10 or 20 weeks of irradiation. Control animals, irradiated without sunscreen protection for the full 30 weeks, sustained severe connective tissue damage that included extensive elastosis, loss of mature collagen, and greatly increased GAGs. Protected animals had only the degree of damage that reflected the weeks of irradiation before sunscreens were applied. As expected, animals irradiated for 20 weeks before sunscreens were applied had considerable photodamage. Nevertheless, during the final 10 weeks of irradiation, with sunscreen protection, a repair zone of new subepidermal collagen was deposited (Fig. 9).

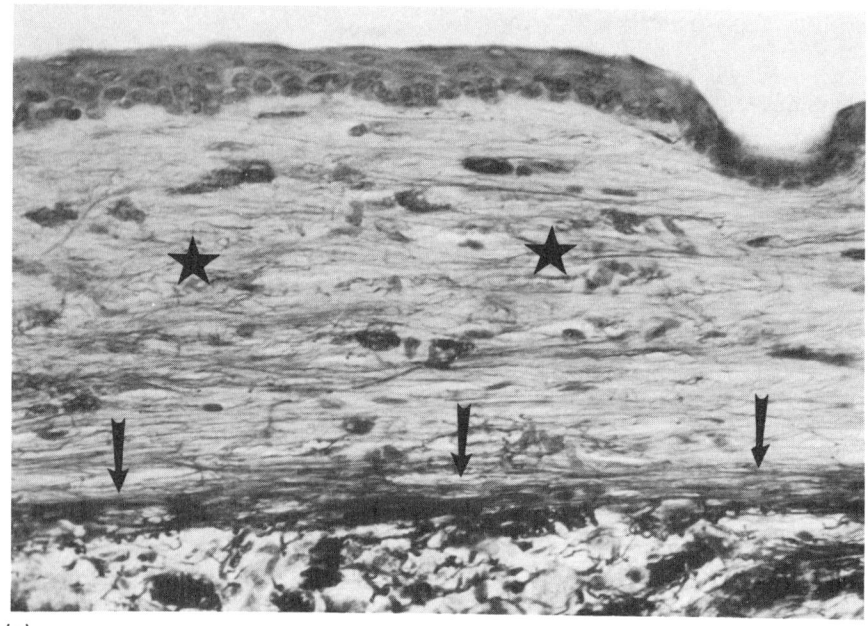

(a)

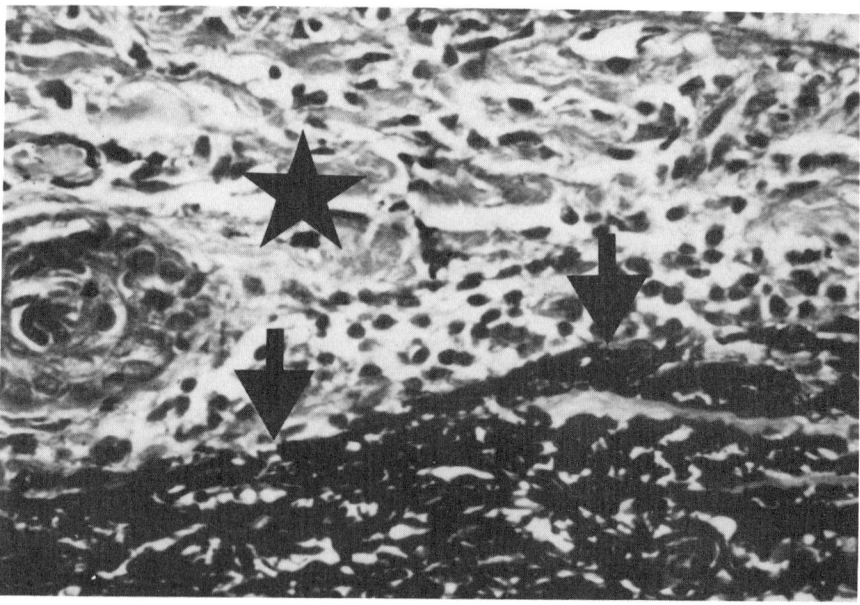

(b)

Figure 8 Post-UV dermal repair is characterized by a large region of new collagen (★) which displaces, downward, the elastosis (→) formed during chronic irradiation. (a) Mouse skin 15 weeks after cessation of irradiation. Note fine new elastic fibers in the repair zone. Luna's stain (X380). (b) Human skin (bald scalp biopsy) after 10 years abstainence from sunbathing. Luna's stain (X380).

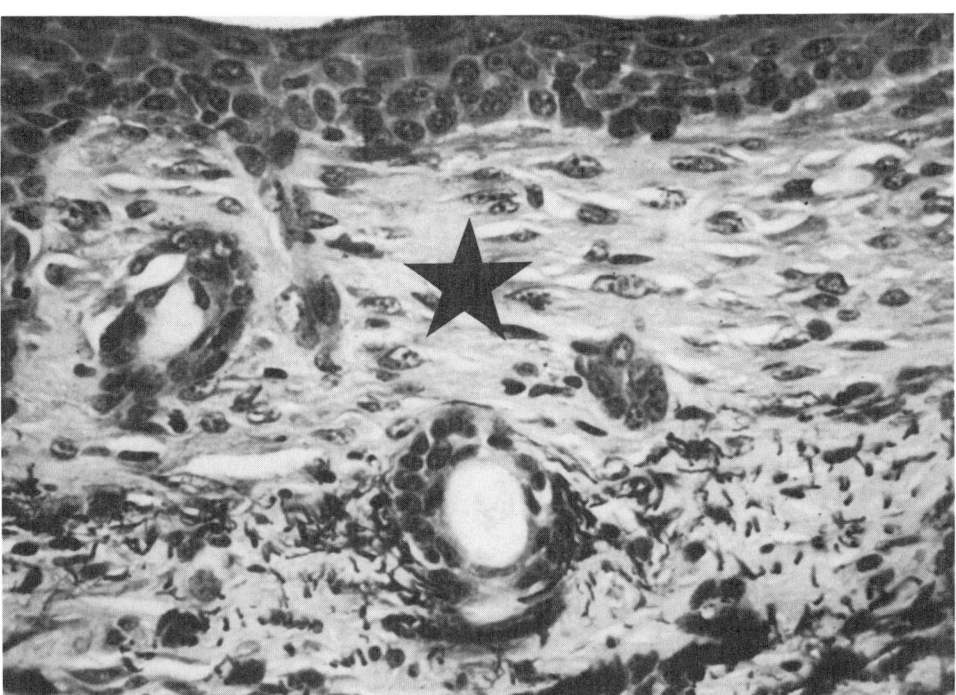

Figure 9 Repair zone (★) in mouse skin irradiated for 30 weeks but protected with an SPF-15 sunscreen for the final 10 weeks. The new collagen has the same staining qualities as the mature collagen in the lower dermis. Luna's stain (×380).

These experiments demonstrated that further damage could be prevented and repair could occur, even in the face of continuing irradiation, once sunscreens were applied. In general, earlier application and higher SPF provided the greatest degree of protection against photoaging. It should be noted that at present, broad-spectrum sunscreens absorb effectively up to approximately 330 nm, providing little protection against a substantial portion of potentially dangerous UVA and none against infrared radiation. The latter cannot be ignored with regard to photoaging. Inseparably linked to sunlight, infrared radiation is perceived as heat. The harmful effect of heat is ancient knowledge (40). Human skin chronically exposed to infrared radiation often develops the condition known as erythema ab igne, with its characteristic mottled pigmentation resulting from damaged, leaking blood vessels. Severe elastic fiber hyperplasia, extending deeply into the dermis, is often present, along with thermal keratoses that are almost identical to those produced by ultraviolet radiation. Experimentally, in a guinea pig model, it has been shown that infrared radiation alone can produce elastosis and can exacerbate the elastosis produced by UVB, adding to photodamage (41).

IV. SUMMARY

In summary, in recent years there has been a growing awareness that many of the so-called attributes of aging skin are, instead, a reflection of environmental assault upon exposed areas of the body. Of special import are the deleterious effects of solar radiation on dermal connective tissue, leading to the visible manifestations of photoaging. Often termed "premature aging," the salient features of the process are distinctly different from those found in normal intrinsic aging.

Experimental studies with animal models have confirmed the notion that the shorter, more energetic portion of the ultraviolet spectrum (UVB) is responsible for much of the dermal connective tissue destruction observed in photoaged skin. More recently, it has been shown that UVA and infrared radiation contribute significantly to photoaging, producing, among other changes, severe elastosis. Because the three broad wavebands are inseparably linked in terrestrial sunlight, all are of concern in the photoaging of human skin.

Photoaged skin damage has been thought to be irreversible. However, our findings indicate that destruction and repair go on simultaneously under continued assault by solar radiation. The balance is shifted toward repair when the radiation stress is relieved. Both epidermis and dermis are capable of moderate self-restoration when exogenous injury ceases, either by avoidance of sunlight or by the use of broad-spectrum, high-SPF sunscreens. Although early protection from sunlight, before severe photodamage occurs, is most desirable, it is deemed advisable to counsel even older persons with photoaged skin to adopt protective measures, thereby allowing repair processes to occur.

REFERENCES

1. Unna, P. *Histopathologie der Hautkrankeiten*, A. Herschwald, Berlin (1894).
2. Dubreuilh, W. Des hyperkeratoses circonscrites. *Ann Derm Syph* (series 3), 7:1158–1204 (1896).
3. Montagna, W. and Carlisle, K. Structural changes in aging human skin. *J. Invest. Dermatol., 73*:47–53 (1979).
4. Plewig, G. and Kligman, A. M. Proliferative activity of the sebaceous glands of the aged. *J. Invest. Dermatol., 70*:314–317 (1978).
5. Kligman, L. H. and Kligman, A. M. Photoaging, *Dermatology in General Medicine*, 3rd edition (T. Fitzpatrick, A. Z. Eisen, K. Wolff, I. M. Freedberg, and K. F. Austen, eds.), McGraw Hill, New York (1986), pp. 1470–1475.
6. Kligman, A. M. Early destructive effects of sunlight on human skin. *J. Am. Med. Assoc., 210*:2377–2380 (1969).

7. Braverman, I. M. and Fonferko, E. Studies in cutaneous aging. I. The elastic fiber network. *J. Invest. Dermatol., 78*:434–444 (1982).

8. Lavker, R. M. Structural alterations in exposed and unexposed aged skin. *J. Invest. Dermatol., 73*:59–66 (1979).

9. Knox, J. M., Cockerell, E. G., and Freeman, R. G. Etiological factors and premature aging. *J. Am. Med. Assoc., 179*:136–142 (1962).

10. Chen, V. L., Fleischmajer, R., Schwartz, E., Palaia, M., and Timpl, R. Immunochemistry of elastotic material in sun-damaged skin. *J. Invest. Dermatol., 87*:334–337 (1986).

11. Kligman, L. H., Akin, F. J., and Kligman, A. M. Sunscreens promote repair of ultraviolet radiation-induced dermal damage. *J. Invest. Dermatol., 81*:98–102 (1983).

12. Lovell, W. W. Ultraviolet irradiation of dermal collagen in vivo. *Trans. St. Johns Hosp. Dermatol. Soc.* (London), *59*:166–174 (1973).

13. Shuster, S. and Bottoms, E. Effect of ultraviolet light on skin collagen. *Nature, 199*:192–193 (1963).

14. Kligman, L. H., Akin, F. J., and Kligman, A. M. The contributions of UVA and UVB to connective tissue damage in hairless mice. *J. Invest. Dermatol., 84*:272–276 (1985).

15. Lavker, R. M. and Kligman, A. M. Chronic heliodermatitis. A morphologic evaluation of chronic actinic damage with emphasis on the role of mast cells. *J. Invest. Dermatol., 90*:325–330 (1988).

16. Werb, Z., Banda, M. J., and Jones, P. A. Degradation of connective tissue matrices by macrophages. I. Proteolysis of elastin, glycoproteins and collagen by proteinases isolated from macrophages. *J. Exp. Med., 152*:1340–1357 (1980).

17. Smith, J. G., Davidson, E. A., Sams, W. M., and Clark, R. D. Alterations in human dermal connective tissue with age and chronic sun damage. *J. Invest. Dermatol., 39*:347–350 (1962).

18. Lovell, C. R., Plastow, S. R., Russell-Jones, R., and Thomas, J. Collagen and elastin in actinic elastosis. *J. Invest. Dermatol., 82*:566a (1984).

19. Bentley, J. P. Aging of collagen. *J. Invest. Dermatol., 73*:80–83 (1979).

20. Yamauchi, M., Woodley, D. T., and Mechanic, G. L. Aging and cross-linking of skin collagen. *Biochem. Biophys Res. Commun., 152*:898–903 (1988).

21. Lavker, R. M., Zheng, P., and Dong, G. Aged skin: a study by light, transmission electron and scanning electron microscopy. *J. Invest. Dermatol., 88*:44–51s (1987).

22. Sams, W. M. and Smith, J. G. The histochemistry of chronically sundamaged skin. *J. Invest. Dermatol., 37*:447–452 (1961).

23. Andrew, W., Behnke, R. H., and Sato, T. Changes with advancing age in the cell population of human dermis. *Gerontologica, 10*:1–19 (1964–65).

24. Kligman, A. M. Perspectives and problems in cutaneous gerontology. *J. Invest. Dermatol., 73*:39–46 (1979).

25. Braverman, I. M. and Fonferko, E. Studies in cutaneous aging II. The microvasculature. *J. Invest. Dermatol., 78*:444–448 (1982).

26. Gilchrest, B. A., Stoff, J. S., and Soter, N. A. Chronologic aging alters the response to UV-induced inflammation in human skin. *J. Invest. Dermatol.*, *79*:11–16 (1982).

27. Urbach, F. Geographic pathology of skin cancers, *The Biologic Effects of Ultraviolet Radiation* (F. Urbach, ed.), Pergamon Press, Oxford (1969), p. 635.

28. Lesnik, R. H., Kligman, L. H., and Kligman, A. M. Chemical and physical injuries to skin cause enlargement of sebaceous glands. *J. Invest. Dermatol.*, *86*:488 (1986).

29. Cole, C. A., Davies, R. E., Forbes, P. D., and D'Aloisio, L. C. Comparison of action spectra for acute cutaneous responses to ultraviolet radiation: Man and albino hairless mouse. *Photochem. Photobiol.*, *37*:623–631 (1983).

30. Kligman, L. H. and Kligman, A. M. Histogenesis and progression of ultraviolet light-induced tumors in hairless mice. *J. Natl. Cancer Inst.*, *67*:1289–1297 (1981).

31. Kligman, L. H., Akin, F. J., and Kligman, A. M. Prevention of ultraviolet damage to the dermis of hairless mice by sunscreens. *J. Invest. Dermatol.*, *78*:181–189 (1982).

32. Bissett, D. L., Hannon, D. P., and Orr, T. V. An animal model of solar-aged skin: histological, physical and visible changes in UV-irradiated hairless mouse skin. *Photochem. Photobiol.*, *46*:367–378 (1987).

33. Sams, W. M., Smith, J. G., and Burk, P. G. The experimental production of elastosis with ultraviolet light. *J. Invest. Dermatol.*, *43*:467–471 (1964).

34. Hirose, R. and Kligman, L. H. An ultrastructural study of ultraviolet-induced elastic fiber damage in hairless mouse skin. *J. Invest. Dermatol.*, *90*:697–702 (1988).

35. Plastow, S. R., Lovell, C. R., and Young, A. R. UVB-induced collagen changes in the skin of the hairless albino mouse. *J. Invest. Dermatol.*, *88*: 145–148 (1987).

36. Schwartz, E., Cruickshank, F. A., Perlish, J. S., and Fleischmajer, R. Alterations in dermal collagen in ultraviolet irradiated hairless mice. *J. Invest. Dermatol.*, *93*:142–146 (1989).

37. Kaidbey, K. H. and Kligman, A. M. The acute effects of longwave ultraviolet radiation on human skin. *J. Invest. Dermatol.*, *72*:253–256 (1979).

38. Gilchrest, B. A., Soter, N. A., Hawk, J. L. M., Barr, R. M., Block, A. K., Hensby, C. N., Mallet, A. I., Greaves, M. W., and Parris, J. A. Histologic changes associated with ultraviolet-A-induced erythema in normal human skin. *J. Am. Acad. Dermatol.*, *9*:213–219 (1983).

39. Kligman, L. H., Kaidbey, K. H., Hitchins, V. M., and Miller, S. A. Long wavelength (>340 nm) ultraviolet-A induced skin damage in hairless mice is dose dependent, *Human Exposure to Ultraviolet Radiation: Risks and Regulation* (W. F. Passchier and B. F. M. Bosnjakovic, eds.), Elsevier Science Publishers B.V. (Biomedical Division) (1987), pp. 77–81.

40. Kligman, L. H. and Kligman, A. M. Reflections on heat. *Br. J. Dermatol.*, *110*:369–375 (1984).

41. Kligman, L. H. Intensification of ultraviolet-induced dermal damage by infrared radiation. *Arch. Dermatol. Res.*, *272*:229–238 (1982).

4
Intrinsic Photoprotection in Human Skin

MADHUKAR A. PATHAK *Harvard Medical School and Massachusetts General Hospital, Boston, Massachusetts*

In this presentation, the photoprotective role of melanin against the acute effects (e.g., sunburn) and the potential long-term risk of actinic changes (e.g., wrinkling or photoaging) and skin cancer (e.g., basal and squamous cell carcinomas and melanomas) is discussed.

To survive the insults of actinic damage, human skin has evolved six defensive mechanisms: (1) the process of keratinization to form a compact, protective layer of stratum corneum; (2) eumelanin pigmentation providing melanin-laden melanosomes that absorb and scatter ultraviolet radiation (UVR); (3) accumulation of carotinoid pigment that acts as a singlet oxygen quencher; (4) UVR-absorbing urocanic acid which undergoes trans–cis isomerization; (5) superoxide dismutase and peroxidase–reductase enzymes that act as scavengers for harmful reactive oxygen species; and (6) error-free DNA repair and replicating mechanism to minimize UVR-induced carcinogenic risk.

The photoprotective role of melanin is attributable to: (1) its biophysical properties (light absorption, attenuation of light by scattering, and dissipation of absorbed energy as heat); (2) its chemical and biochemical properties to act as a free radical scavenger and electron exchange polymer in the oxidation-reduction reaction; and (3) its ability to act as a pseudo dismutase and a scavenger of superoxide anions generated by UVR.

I. INTRODUCTION

Human skin is much more than an inert body sheath. The skin is uniquely structured to function as a major barrier to protect the underlying organs against the ravages of the environment. This multilayered cellular barrier endowed with cohesive stratum corneum not only prevents the loss of essential body fluids but regulates thermal homeostasis in both warm and cold climates. It retards the entrance of potentially toxic agents and the invasion of pathogenic microorganisms. It protects itself and the underlying organs against mechanical forces and the harmful effects of ultraviolet radiation (UVR). In this presentation, my comments shall be limited to the photoprotective role of melanin, an important chromophore of human skin that protects it against the harmful effects of UVR. Human skin color is a composite of red (oxyhemoglobin), blue (reduced hemoglobin), yellow (carotenoids and flavins), and brown (melanin). While the ranges of normal skin color (from white, light tan, yellow-brown, brown, and black) are the result of admixtures of these four colors, the human race with regard to their basic skin color can be divided into the three basic colors of white, brown, and black as a result of variations in the amount and distribution of melanin in epidermal cells. These three basic colors have further variations: (a) white and pink-white such as observed in Scandinavians, Norwegians, Anglo-Saxon, Celtics, etc.; (b) light tan in fair-skinned French, Germans, Northern Italians, Greeks, etc.; (c) yellowish tan in fair-skinned Japanese, Chinese, Amerindians, etc.; (d) brown in dark-skinned East Indians, Hispanics, Portuguese, etc.; and (e) black in Africans, Australian Aborigenes, black Americans, etc.

This impressive variation is due largely to genetic and acquired differences (environmental influences such as solar radiation, proximity to the equator, etc.) in the amount and distribution of epidermal melanin pigmentation. In all races, skin devoid of melanogenic activity of melanocytes is unquestionably white. The other major factor influencing normal skin color is blood content in vessels of the superficial dermal plexus, which imparts a pink or reddish hue. The infinite number of hues observed in different races of the world are highly influenced by the spectral quality of light and also from the intensity of light reaching the skin and the human eye. There are two major types of integumentary melanins: (1) brown-black eumelanin, and (2) yellow-red pheomelanin. Both types are formed by the action of tyrosinase. In melanocytes, tyrosinase converts tyrosine to dopa and dopa to dopaquinone, which is then cyclized and oxidized to form eumelanin. This melanin is considered to be primarily a polyindolequinone. Pheomelanin, the term used for yellow-red macromolecular pigments, is formed by cysteinyl dopa oxidation products resulting from the nucleophilic addition of the amino acid cysteine (or other related sulfhydryl compounds such as glutathione) to dopaquinone in the presence of tyrosinase. In pheomelanin, 5S-cysteinyl dopa is a major monomer unit (1). Pheomelanin is photolabile and does not appear to have photoprotective properties. This brief review focuses on the photoprotective role of eumelanin against the acute effects (e.g., sunburn and phototoxicity) and the potential long-term risk of actinic changes (wrinkling and premature aging of skin) and premalignancies and malignancies (solar kertosis, basal and squamous cell carcinomas, and even melanomas) that are caused by exposure of human skin to solar radiation.

II. NATURAL DEFENSES OF SKIN AGAINST SUNLIGHT

One of the most important of the many diversified functions of skin is the protection of internal organs and the integument itself against the acute and chronic damaging effects of solar radiation. To survive the insults of actinic damage resulting from direct (intentional sunbathing) or indirect sun exposure (unavoidable outdoor exposure), human skin has evolved six basic defensive mechanisms (2–7).

1. The process of keratinization leading to the formation of compact and cohesive horny cell layer (stratum corneum) of varying thickness containing ultraviolet-absorbing proteins (amino acids of keratins); the compact horny layer not only absorbs UVR to prevent its transmission to the viable cells of epidermis but also attenuates the impinging radiation by scattering.

2. The process of genetically controlled constitutive melanin pigmentation in melanocytes involving the formation, melanization, and transfer of melanosomes from melanocytes to keratinocytes. Melanin in epidermal keratinocytes exists in a colloidal (amorphous) form and in an organelle form (melanosomes); both act as a UV-absorbing optical filter and a free-radical scavenger to provide a shield to nuclear DNA of keratinocytes and the dermal proteins, collagen and elastin, against UVR-induced harmful alterations (e.g., formation of pyrimidine photoadducts or dimers and cross-links in proteins) (3,6,8).

3. The preferential accumulation of carotenoid pigment (β-carotene) in subcutaneous tissue allows this biochrome to diffuse and to enrich both the epidermal and dermal cells to act as a membrane stabilizer and a quencher against the damaging forms of reactive O_2 species (singlet oxygen or $^1O_2$, superoxide anion or O_2^-, hydroxy radical or ·OH, etc.) generated by UVR.

4. The formation and accumulation of urocanic acid, the deaminated product of histidine in the epidermis, which by virtue of its ability to undergo cis-trans isomerization and oxidation reaction protects the viable cells of the epidermis against actinic damage (5).

5. The presence of superoxide dismutase (SOD) and glutathione peroxidase-reductase enzyme system in the epidermis acting as selective scavengers for inactivating the reactive forms of O_2 (superoxide anion or O_2^-) generated by UVR and protecting cell membranes from lipoprotein damage resulting from lipid-peroxidation reaction. These two enzymes also protect the epidermal and dermal proteins (keratin, elastin, and collagen) against

the cross-linking reaction resulting from the harmful effects of reactive oxygen generated by UVR (6,7).

6. The excision repair capacity of cutaneous cells to appropriately repair UVR-induced damage to DNA by an error-free DNA replicating mechanism in order to minimize the potential for UV-induced skin carcinogenesis. Xeroderma pigmentosum or XP, an autosomal recessive disease, serves as the prototype in which the defective excision repair due to altered endonuclease activity and diminished photoreactivation repair in the XP cell strain leads to an early onset of neoplastic changes (5,9).

Although these six defensive mechanisms in mammalian skin are important and compliment each other, normal human skin of most individuals has two major defensive barriers that play a significant role in protection against the harmful effects of UVR. These include: (a) the compact multicell layer of the stratum corneum, and (b) the presence of the melanin filter in the viable cells of epidermis that shields the nuclear DNA from harmful alterations. Of these two barriers to UVR, the melanin filter is the most important, inasmuch as humans with normal stratum corneum but without melanin (e.g., albinos or amelanotic skin of vitiligo patients) succumb to repeated UV exposures with early onset of chronic solar damage (actinic elastosis or dermatoheliosis) and skin cancer despite the capacity of the albino or vitiliginous skin to respond normally by the process of hyperplasia and subsequent thickening of the stratum corneum. The central factor in assessing the relative importance of natural defenses of skin against UVR exposure is the presence or absence of melanized epidermis (i.e., brown or black skin) and the genetic capacity of the individual to develop melanized epidermis (light, moderate, or dark tan).

Because of limitations of space, only the photoprotective property of eumelanin (brown-black) will be discussed.

III. PHOTOPROTECTIVE ROLE OF MELANIN

Not all people in the world share an equal risk for the development of dermatoheliosis (photoaging or changes in connective tissue components of the dermis, including the vascular system, collagen and elastin tissue leading to wrinkling and thining of skin) and development of skin cancer. We will first document nature's well-controlled experiment to illustrate the unique photoprotective role of melanin.

The world population contains over 2.5 billion nonwhite people (individuals of Skin Types IV, V, and VI) whose skin on unexposed parts of the body (e.g., buttock) is brown or black due to the presence of a large amount of melanin. Their sun-exposed skin is well pigmented. These individuals live in hot, sunny regions, but are significantly resistant to the deleterious effects of UVR, while the remaining white population in excess of one billion living in Europe, the United Kingdom, North and South America, South Africa, Australia, etc., have white skin in these unexposed areas due to a low amount of melanin and exhibit all the acute and chronic problems associated with exposure to sunlight (e.g., sunburn, keratoses, dermatoheliosis or changes associated with photoaging, such as wrinkling, freckling, lentigenes, and telangiectasia, and skin cancer of habitually exposed skin areas). The nearly 700 million people of the Middle East (Saudi Arabia, Lebanon, Iran, etc.), India, and Pakistan, although classified as Caucasians, have moderately brown skin of unexposed areas and are not easily susceptible to sun-induced damage (dermatoheliosis) even though the intensity of harmful UVR in this region is significantly high throughout the year (5).

Phenotypic characteristics associated with skin cancer in well-documented studies (9,10) include humans with a fair complexion, light eyes, and light hair color (usually individuals with blond or red hair, blue eyes, and freckles) and who sunburn easily and repeatedly, and exhibit a poor ability to tan. Individuals of Celtic descent (e.g., Scottish, Irish, and Welsh) are particularly vulnerable to skin cancer. The highest incidences of skin tumors are seen among the Anglo-Saxon and Celtic population in such areas as Queensland, Australia and Arizona and New Mexico in the United States. By way of contrast, skin cancer is relatively rare in brown and darkly pigmented people; basal cell epitheliomas are uncommon while the squamous cell carcinomas, if observed, generally occur on lower extremities and do not appear related to UVR. The incidence of melanoma in the non-white world population is also very low (less than 0.9 per 100,000) compared to an average incidence of 4.5 per 100,000 in whites. In Australia, the incidence of melanoma in the fair-skinned population is 25.0 per 100,000 (9,10).

In pigmented persons, a unique light-absorbing and UV-filtering system is usually distributed as a supranuclear cap of melanin-laden melanosomes in the basal and suprabasal cells to minimize the impact of photons on viable cells of the epidermis (3,5,8). In humans of Skin Types IV, V, and VI, active epidermal melanin units (melanocytes producing and transferring melanosomes to keratinocytes) provide a front line of defense against UV and visible radiation. The white population possesses a lesser amount of this protective filter (eumelanin), while brown- and black-skinned people are endowed with a significant amount of melanin that acts as a major barrier to the penetration of harmful UV rays. The protective role of melanin in the epidermis is attributable to its presence in two distinct forms: (a) particulate form referred to as melanosomes, and (b) nonparticulate, colloidal or amorphous form (3,8). In the stratum corneum, most of the melanin is usually in a nonparticulate amorphous form, although in certain brown- and black-skinned individuals one will find a few melanosomes in a particulate form scattered randomly in nonviable horny cells. The amorphous form of melanin is derived from the particulate form of melansomes by the

process of enzymatic degradation due to the presence of hydrolytic and proteolytic enzymes associated with melanosome complexes or in the outer membrane
layer of these discrete organelles. This amorphous form of the melanin, which is
primarily rich in polyindolequinones, undergoes rapid oxidation reaction and is
usually manifested as immediate pigment darkening (IPD) reaction when the
skin is exposed to solar radiation or to UVA radiation (320–400 nm) from artificial light sources (11). This IPD reaction, to a limited extent, constitutes a
photoprotective mechanism and is usually more prominent in light- or dark-
skinned individuals of Skin Types III through VI. The remainder of the viable
epidermal cells (basal and malpighian cells) contain melanin-laden melanosomes
in particulate form. The particulate form of melanin not only absorbs but also
scatters the impinging UVR.

IV. MODE OF PROTECTION BY MELANIN

The photoprotective role of melanin is accomplished by the physical and biochemical properties of the polymer outlined below:

 1. A chemically prepared melanin derived from the auto-oxidation of 3,4-
dihydroxyphenylalanine (dopa), and melanin isolated from human hair,
melanoma cells, and pigmented skin of black guinea pigs is a heteropolymer
(random) consisting of several different monomer units including indole 5,6-
quinone and coupled by various bond types; such a polymer reveals significant
absorption characteristics in UV (200–400 nm) and visible spectrum (400–760
nm). It can also act as an effective filter to screen out harmful UVR. Melanized
epidermis acts as a cloak to shield the viable cells of the epidermis and dermis by
reducing the transmission of damaging UVB and UVA radiation. This is best
documented in nature's ongoing experiment in humans living in the equatorial
regions of the world. Sun-induced nonmelanoma skin cancer on the habitually
exposed areas of the face and upper extremities is very rare in the Blacks of
equatorial Africa and Aborigenes of Australia, New Guinea, and southern India
living in tropical areas with high solar UVB and UVA flux; on the other hand,
Black albinos living in South Africa or fair-skinned Australians living in proximity to Australian Aborigenes develop solar keratoses and skin cancer at an early
age (9,10).

 2. There is an apparent inverse relationship between skin sensitivity (reactivity) to UVR and melanin content. The 300-nm transmittance of full-thickness
suction-separated epidermis including the basal cell layer varies two to three
orders of magnitude from a fair-skinned Caucasian of Skin Type I to a darkly
pigmented Skin Type V or VI with brown or black skin. Table 1 provides the
laboratory determined values for minimal erythema response (MED) in over 100
individuals represented by a minimum of 10 individuals in each skin type ranging
from Types I through VI. Richly melanized skin exhibits higher MED values

Table 1   MED Values in Normal Individuals of Skin Types I Through VI Based
on Sunburn and Suntanning History

Skin type	Unexposed buttock skin	Sun sensitivity and pigment response[a]	UVB MED (MJ/cm^2)
I	White	Always burn easily, tan little or none	20–30
II	White	Always burn easily, tan minimally with difficulty	25–35
III	White	Always burn moderately, tan average (light brown)	30–50
IV	Light brown	Burn minimally, exhibit IPD, tan easily (moderate brown)	50–75
V	Moderate brown	Burn with difficulty and minimally, exhibit intense IPD and tan profusely	60–90
VI	Dark brown, black	Insensitive, never burn, tan profusely	100–200

[a]Based on first 30 to 45 minutes of sun exposure after winter season or without previous sun exposure.
IPD = immediate pigment darkening.

than poorly melanized skin. When compared with amelanotic skin of albinos, the sun protection factor (SPF) value for melanin in the unexposed skin of the lower back and buttock ranges from 2 in individuals of Skin Type II to about 6 in individuals of Skin Type VI. However, it should be recognized that protection of skin against exposures to UVR is not only due to the increasing content of melanin through neomelanogenesis but also due to epidermal cell hyperplasia. The relative degree of UV-induced photoprotection offered by neomelanogenesis versus epidermal-cell hyperplasia depends upon the wavelengths in question. For UVB wavelengths, both the increased production of melanin and hyperplasia, offer effective photoprotection; but for UVA and visible wavelengths, melanin is the only major epidermal chromophore. Whereas both UVA and UVB radiation induce neomelanogenesis, there is relatively greater epidermal-cell hyperplasia after UVB. Thus, more pigment may be transformed to the stratum corneum leading to greater photoprotection when skin is exposed to UVB rather than to UVA radiation. UVA-induced tanning may be less protective against UVB radiation than UVB-induced tanning.

The second most important property by which melanin exerts photoprotection involves scattering. Unlike absorption, scattering is not only dependent upon the wavelength impinging on the skin, but also depends considerably upon the physical size of the scattering structure. Melanin-laden melanosomes, present as supranuclear caps in keratinocytes, attenuate the impinging UVR by scattering. This scattering involves any process within the epidermis that deflects electromagnetic radiation from a straight line path and results in the attenuation of radiation. This increases the total absorbing path through which the photons of UV must pass. For melanin particles with dimensions of the order of wavelength of the UVR (300 nm), the impinging photons may be scattered according to the Rayleigh relation (scattering is inversely proportional to the fourth power of the incident light such that the shortest wavelengths are more strongly scattered). Maximum scattering occurs when the wavelength of light approaches the particle size. For particles of melanosomes larger in size than the wavelength of the incident light (e.g., melanosomes which are 0.6–1.0 μM in size), the scattering relationship becomes quite complex, but nonetheless dominates in deviating the course of penetrating photons. The UV photons in brown and darkly pigmented skin are significantly attenuated by scattering in a forward direction.

3. Melanin also protects skin cells against the harmful effects of UVR and visible radiation through the process of absorption and dissipation of the absorbed energy as heat. In this regard, it is of interest to note that during the summer months one sees more of fair-skinned individuals (Types I-III) sunbathing on beaches than dark-skinned individuals (Types V-VI). In contrast to fair-skinned individuals endowed with a low concentration of melanin, who enjoy sunbathing without any discomfort, the high concentration of melanin in the darkly pigmented skin makes sunbathing a less enjoyable event. The heat generated in the skin by absorption of radiant energy causes discomfort to the pigmented individual. In this regard, it is of interest to point out the hypothesis of McGinnes and Procter (12) and McGinnes et al. (13) that melanin in the epidermal cells may serve as a device by which it may convert the energy of the excited states into heat by a phenomenon known as photo-phonon conversion. This hypothesis implies that a melanin polymer can act as an amorphous semiconductor in which the coupling of phonons (i.e., the vibrational modes of melanin polymer to its excited electronic states) plays a major role in the dissipation of energy absorbed from the impinging UVR.

4. An additional way by which melanin exerts a photoprotective effect in vivo is by way of utilizing the absorbed energy into a harmless photochemical reaction. Dermatologists and photobiologists are familiar with the phenomenon of immediate pigment darkening or IPD reaction (11,14) in which the exposed skin becomes darker during irradiation. In this reaction, the absorbed UVR energy (300–360 nm) induces immediate oxidation in the melanin polymer through the generation of semiquinone free radicals (14,15). Although recent observations on IPD reaction reported by Honigsmann et al. (16) suggest that this photochemical event does not provide a protective effect on the degree of sunburn reaction or on the induction of epidermal DNA damage in the form of thymine dimers, one must be very cautious in leading to conclusions based on

negative findings. DNA damage by UVB radiation (e.g., formation of thymine dimers) is generally not an oxygen-dependent oxidative reaction; it results from the direct absorption of photons and does not involve reactive oxygen. Oxidative damage is distinct (e.g., membrane lipid peroxidation, oxidation of membrane-bound cytochrome P-450, etc.) and is mediated by the production of reactive oxygen species ($^1O_2$, O_2^-, $\cdot OH$, etc.) (17). IPD reaction will undoubtedly minimize such an oxidative damage in epidermal cells.

5. One of the important properties of melanin by which it exerts photoprotection in human skin is its ability to act as a free radical scavenger for minimizing the harmful effects of other free radicals generated by UVR. Melanin exists in human skin as a stable free radical. As a stable free radical, melanin by its ability to undergo immediate oxidation and reduction reaction, can act as a biologic electron exchange polymer and minimize the impact of the impinging photons on the other vulnerable cell constituents (e.g., cell membranes, oxidative enzymes, such as SOD, etc.). The free radicals in melanin are quite stable and the unpaired electrons seem to be limited to localized regions of the polymer and are stabilized by a large number of resonance structures within the polymer. Because of the unpaired electrons in the melanin polymer, it may in effect serve as a one-dimensional semi-conductor, where any bound protons serve as electron traps. A free flow of charge in the form of electrons is then possible through the melanin (18). It is known that UV irradiation increases the unpaired spin concentration in biological tissue such as skin; presumably an internal oxidative-reduction reaction is occurring with the production of some new radicals (14,15). The trapping of free radicals which could disrupt the metabolism of living cells is feasible in the presence of stable free radicals in melanin polymer. It appears that melanin can also act as a scavenger of superoxide anion (O_2^-) or $\cdot OH$ radicals. In this regard, it acts as a pseudo-dismutase. Recent studies definitely indicate that UVR generates free radicals and reactive oxygen species [singlet oxygen ($^1O_2$ and O_2^-)], both *in vitro* and *in vivo* (6,7,17). The consequences of free radical generation by UVR to a living system such as human skin are numerous and complex. Free radicals and reactive oxygen species can induce: (a) strand session, (b) DNA-protein cross-links, (c) cross-linking of proteins (e.g., in collagen and elastin), (d) inactivation of enzymes, (e) peroxidation of membrane lipids, and (f) oxidation of sulfhydryl groups causing alterations in the structural and functional state of proteins, etc. These reactive oxygen species are known to be toxic to the viability of cells. Melanin-containing cells are certainly less vulnerable to such oxidative effects of reactive oxygen.

V. SUMMARY

In this presentation, the photoprotective role of melanin in human skin against the acute effects (e.g., sunburn) and the potential long-term risks of actinic changes (wrinkling and premature aging of the skin) and premalignancies and malignancies (solar kertosis, basal and squamous cell carcinomas, and even melanomas) are discussed. Melanin, present in the epidermis in a particulate form as melanosomes and in an amorphous form as colloidal melanin provides protection to the viable cells of epidermis and dermis in one or more of the following forms: (a) it acts as a filter to screen out harmful UV; (b) it absorbs UVR and dissipates the absorbed energy into heat; (c) melanin-laden melanosomes, which are bigger than the wavelengths of UVR impinging on the skin, scatter and attenuate UVR; (d) melanin as a stable free radical and as a biological electron-exchange polymer acts as a scavenger or quencher of unpaired electrons in reactions involving oxidations and reductions; and (e) melanin also acts as a pseudo dismutase and a scavenger of superoxide anions generated by UVA radiation.

ACKNOWLEDGMENT

This work was supported by NIH grant 5-R01-CA-05003-29 awarded by the US National Cancer Institute, Department of Health, Education, and Welfare, Bethesda, MD.

REFERENCES

1. Wick, M. M. Melanin: structure and properties, in *Brown Melanoderma*, (T. B. Fitzpatrick, M. M. Wick, and K. Toda, eds.), Tokyo, University of Tokyo Press (1986), pp. 37–44.
2. Pathak, M. A. The role of natural photoprotective agents in human skin, in *Sunlight and Man* (M. A. Pathak, L. C. Harber, M. Seiji, and A. Kukita, eds.), University Tokyo Press, Tokyo, (1974), pp. 725–750.
3. Pathak, M. A., Jimbow, K., Szabo, G., and Fitzpatrick, T. B. Sunlight and melanin pigmentation, in *Photochemical and Photobiological Reviews* (K. C. Smith, ed.), New York, Plenum Press (1976), pp. 211–239.
4. Pathak, M. A. Reactive oxygen species and free radicals in sunlight-induced skin reactions. *J. Am. Oil Chem. Soc., 64*:630 (1987).
5. Pathak, M. A., Fitzpatrick, T. B., Greiter, F. J., and Kraus, E. W. Preventive treatment of sunburn, dermatoheliosis, and skin cancer with sun protective agents, in *Dermatology in General Medicine*, 3rd ed. (T. B. Fitzpatrick, A. Z. Eisen, K. Wolff, et al., eds.), New York, McGraw-Hill, (1987), pp. 1507–1522.
6. Carraro, C. and Pathak, M. A. Characterization of superoxide dismutase from mammalian skin epidermis. *J. Invest. Dermatol., 90*:31–36 (1988).
7. Carraro, C. and Pathak, M. A. Studies in the nature of in vitro and in vivo photosensitization reactions by psoralens and porphyrins. *J. Invest. Dermatol., 90*:267–275 (1988).
8. Pathak, M. A. Epidermal melanin pigmentation stimulated by ultraviolet radiation and psoralens, in *Brown Melanoderma*, (T. B. Fitzpatrick, M. M. Wick, and K. Toda, eds.), Tokyo, University Tokyo Press, (1986), pp. 97–114.

9. Urbach, F. Photocarcinogenesis, in *The Science of Photomedicine*, (J. D. Regan and J. A. Parrish, eds.), New York, Plenum Press (1982), pp. 261–292.

10. Kopf, A. W., Kripke, M. L., and Stern, R. S. Sun and malignant melanoma. *J. Am. Acad. Dermatol.*, *11*:674–684 (1984).

11. Pathak, M. A. Immediate and delayed pigmentary and other cutaneous responses to solar UVA radiation (320–400 nm), in *The Biological Effects of UVA Radiation* (F. Urbach and R. W. Gange, eds.), New York, Praeger Publishers (1986), pp. 156–167.

12. McGinness, J. E. and Proctor, P. H. The importance of the fact that melanin is black. *J. Theor. Biol.*, *39*:677 (1973).

13. McGinness, M. C., Corry, P., and Procter, P. Amorphous semiconductor switching in melanin. *Science, 183*:853–855 (1974).

14. Pathak, M. A. Photobiology of melanogenesis: Biophysical aspects. In *Advances of Biology of Skin; the Pigmentary System*, Vol. 8 (W. Montagna and F. Hu, eds.), Oxford, Pergamon Press, (1967), pp. 387–420.

15. Pathak, M. A. and Stratton, K. A study of the free radicals in human skin before and after exposure to light. *Arch. Biochem. Biophys., 123*:468–476 (1968).

16. Hongismann, H., Schuler, G., Aberer, W., Romam, N., and Wolff, K. Immediate pigment darkening phenomenon: A reevaluation of its mechanisms. *J. Invest. Dermatol., 87*:648–652 (1986).

17. Pathak, M. A. and Carraro, C. Reactive oxygen species in cutaneous photosensitivity reactions in porphyrias and PUVA photochemotherapy and in melanin pigmentation, in *The Biological Role of Reactive Oxygen Species in Skin*, (O. Hayaishi, S. Imamura, and Y. Miyachi, eds.), Tokyo, University of Tokyo Press (1987), pp. 75–94.

18. Mason, H. S., Ingram, D. J. E., and Allen, B. The free radical property of melanins. *Arch. Biochem. Biophys., 86*:225–230 (1960).

5

Sunscreen Use and Nonmelanoma Skin Cancer

ROBERT S. STERN   *Harvard Medical School and Beth Israel Hospital, Boston, Massachusetts*

I. INTRODUCTION

This chapter will review the evidence that sunlight is the principal etiologic factor in the development of nonmelanoma skin cancer (NMSC) in humans. It will then present evidence that regular use of sunscreens should reduce the risk of nonmelanoma skin cancer.

At least eight factors influence the effectiveness of sunscreens in reducing the risk of NMSC. Those determiners to be considered here include:

1. The relationship between dose of sunlight to which an individual is exposed and the risk of NMSC
2. The action spectrum for the development of NMSC
3. The absorption characteristics of sunscreens
4. Life-time exposure patterns to sunlight
5. Possible differences in the individual's susceptibility to the carcinogenic effects of sunlight at different periods during a lifetime and as a consequence of prior exposures to sunlight and other carcinogens
6. Changes in exposure habits that occur as a result of sunscreen use
7. Loss of acclimatization that may occur as a result of sunscreen use
8. The possible toxicity of sunscreens

The relative importance of each of these factors in determining an individual's risk of NMSC is likely to vary with age. Further, there are likely to be interactions between each of these factors which make it difficult to estimate precisely the utility of sunscreens for a particular individual for a given period of time. As an illustration of the possible substantial protective effect of a sunscreen, the assumptions and results of an analysis that predicted risk reduction for NMSC with the use of sunscreens in childhood use will be reviewed (1).

II. RELATION OF SUN EXPOSURE TO RISK OF NMSC

Perhaps the best evidence for the association between cumulative solar exposure and the risk of NMSC comes from the elegant federal surveys conducted by Scotto and his colleagues at the National Cancer Institute (2). These surveys attempted to ascertain all incident cases of nonmelanoma skin cancers in eight geographic areas which vary substantially in their latitude, altitude, and average cloud cover and hence the amount of sunlight and ultraviolet exposure per year. These incidence data combined with various measurements of exposure form the core of specific mathematical models which estimate the dose/risk relationship between sunlight, ultraviolet exposure, and NMSC. Some of these models are considered in greater detail below.

The federal data document four points. First, these data clearly show that the incidence of NMSC is higher in areas with greater annual ultraviolet B (UVB, 290–320 nm) insolation. Second, the incidence of NMSC increases with age; and third, this age-related increase in risk in each geographic area is greater than would be accounted for if prior cumulative exposure alone were the sole determinate of the risk of NMSC. Finally, these data indicate that increased exposure to UVB radiation is more strongly associated with the risk of squamous cell carcinoma (SCC) than of basal cell carcinoma (BCC).

These four facts are illustrated by a comparison of UVB insolation and incidence rates for Minneapolis, Minnesota and Atlanta, Georgia. The annual UVB insolation for Atlanta is 50% greater than it is in Minneapolis. The age-adjusted incidence rate of BCC in Atlanta is more than twice that in Minneapolis. The age-adjusted incidence rate for SCC in Atlanta is approximately four times that of the rate for Minneapolis. For SCC in Minneapolis, the risk for individuals 55 to 64 years old is only one-fifth that for individuals only 20 years older. For BCC, the rate for 55 to 64 year olds is approximately 40% the rate for those 20 years older.

Basing their work on incidence data from the federal survey, a number of investigators have attempted to determine the extent to which the increase or decrease in sun exposure influences the risk of NMSC. By basing calculations on the action spectrum for DNA damage and on the results of animal experiments, it has been determined that UVB solar radiation waves in the 290–320 nm range are the most dangerously efficient wavelengths with respect to mutagenesis and carcinogenesis (3–5). Therefore, most of these models have related UVB exposure rather than total sunlight exposure to NMSC risk.

At least three groups have attempted to quantify the relationship between change in lifetime UVB dosage and the risk of NMSC (6-8). All three groups used measurements of UVB in various geographic areas to determine exposure and to relate these measurements to age-specific incidence rates in these locations. In general, these models assume that incidence at a given time depends on cumulative dose and that an individual's annual dose is likely to be approximately constant over a lifetime's residence in a given geographic area.

Given the similar data used to fit the models and the comparable assumptions these models make, it is not surprising that these studies yield relatively comparable results. These models predict that a 1.0% increase in UVB lifetime exposure will increase the lifetime risk of NMSC by more than 1.0%.

Further, the increase in incidence of SCC with increasing UVB exposure is greater than that observed for BCC. Also, increasing exposure for males results in a greater increase in incidence than in females. For example, using Caucasian subjects only, Fears and Scotto predicted a 1.0% increase in UVB exposure would increase the incidence of BCC in males by 1.3 to 2.6 percent and by 1.1 to 2.1 percent for females (7). For SCC, a 1.0% increase UVB exposure would increase the incidence of these tumors by 2.1 to 4.1% for males and 2.2 to 4.3% for females.

Evidence from animal experiments suggests that the development of NMSC is a multistage process. At least one study suggests that only initiation and not promotion is dependent upon UVB exposure (9). These findings suggest that exposure received early in life may be a more important determinant of lifetime NMSC risk than exposure received in later years. In addition, for many individuals, the pattern of exposure to sunlight and hence UVB may vary over their lifetimes.

As detailed below, using a multistage model permits assessment of the effect of varying patterns of exposure to UVB on the risk of NMSC. Using such a multistage model, we previously estimated the risk reduction for NMSC which can be accomplished with varying periods and degrees of sunscreen use during childhood (1). Predictions based on this model are detailed below.

III. ACTION SPECTRUM: SPECTRA OF NMSC

The action spectrum for the mutagenic effects of ultraviolet radiation and its carcinogenic effects are likely to be similar. Therefore, of the wavelengths of light that reach the Earth's surface, UVB radiation is by far the most mutagenic and carcinogenic (3,4). For example, after allowance is made for transmission of UVB radiation through the skin, one joule of 300 nm UVB radiation has more than a 1000-fold greater carcinogenic effect than the same dose of 330 nm radiation.

IV. ABSORPTION CHARACTERISTIC OF SUNSCREENS

Sunscreens containing para amino benzoic acid (PABA) and PABA esters have relatively constant absorption throughout the UVB spectrum. Given the action spectrum for erythema and carcinogenesis, and the absorption characteristics of sunscreens that contain these agents, it is likely that the protective factor offered by a sunscreen against carcinogenic radiation at least equals the protective factor calculated for erythema for that sunscreen. For example, a sunscreen with an SPF of 15 should absorb more than 90% of the UVB radiation responsible for carcinogenesis as it is applicable to an individual of a given age and history of exposure.

Given the relationship of dose to risk of NMSC, the action spectrum for cutaneous carcinogenesis and the absorption characteristics of sunscreens, one would therefore assume that habitual use of a sunscreen with a SPF of 15 or greater throughout life should prevent the occurrence of most NMSCs that are attributed to sun exposure. A consideration of additional factors reveals why the use of sunscreens by some individuals has not led to any apparent substantial decreases in the incidence of NMSC risk to date.

V. VARIATION IN UVB EXPOSURE WITH AGE AND
BETWEEN INDIVIDUALS

With the exception of our earlier work (1), most models that relate NMSC incidence to UVB dosage assume constant exposure throughout a lifetime. Our analysis, on the other hand, assumed that the quantity of UVB exposure varied over a person's lifetime. For most individuals, there are more frequent opportunities for outdoor activity and hence sun exposure during childhood than for the same individuals as adults. For such individuals, initiating sunscreen use after childhood would decrease lifetime UVB exposure by only a small fraction. For example, if we assume the average child (to age 18 years) receives three times as much UVB per year as an adult, if the individual now age 36 years had used sunscreens faithfully for the last 18 years (the time during which such sunscreens were widely available), the maximum reduction in total UVB incidence would total only 20% even if SPF 15 sunscreen had been used throughout this interval.

VI. DIFFERENCES IN RISK WITH EXPOSURE AS A
FUNCTION OF AGE

DeGruij et al.'s work with mice (9) strongly suggests that initiation of NMSC is dependent upon UV-B dose but that once initiation has occurred, the chances of tumor development depend largely on time rather than subsequent exposure. Our multistage model also predicts that some stages of tumor development are only time dependent and are not dependent on exposure. If this observation pertains to humans, it could be argued that the use of sunscreens after a sufficient dose of UVB had been received to initiate tumor formation would have little impact on the subsequent risk of NMSC. Therefore, the use of sunscreens later in life might provide little protection against cancer compared with the effect of such use earlier.

Alternatively, it has been observed that actinic keratoses tend to progress with sun exposure and to regress when sun exposure is halted. These observations suggest that UVB radiation is not only an initiator but also a promoter of NMSC. Unfortunately, data to determine at what period in relation to the development of a tumor the presumed promotional effects of UVB radiation are most important are not now available.

The lack of knowledge about when UVB is most important as a promoter does not permit a prediction of whether using a sunscreen in middle or old age might be more effective in reducing the risk of NMSC. However, the behavior of actinic keratoses in response to sun exposure suggests that the promotion of NMSC by UVB may come as a late stage. If this is the case, sun protection in persons with sun-damaged skin and with histories of malignant or premalignant tumors might be especially important.

VII. ESTIMATING RISK REDUCTION FOR NMSC BY THE USE OF SUNSCREENS

Basing our work on the dose/risk relationship and action spectrum of NMSC discussed above, we developed a multistage model of carcinogenesis which permitted us to estimate the effects of varying periods of sunscreen use during childhood on the lifetime risk of NMSC. Based on epidemiologic data, our model indicates that there are two dose-dependent stages in the development of NMSC and three additional time-dependent stages for males and two such stages for females. This model permitted estimation of the extent to which the reductions in dose achieved by the use of sunscreen protection during various intervals of childhood might reduce the risk of NMSC.

In our base case analysis, we estimated that exposure per year in childhood was three times the exposure per year as adults. We assumed that in actual use, regular application of a SPF 15 sunscreen would reduce absorbed UV-B radiation by approximately 85%. In our base case analysis we further assumed that one of the dose-dependent stages occurs in childhood (i.e., *initiation*) and the other dose-dependent stage later in life, (i.e., *promotion*).

Under these assumptions, we estimate that regular use of a SPF 15 sunscreen to age 18 years would reduce the lifetime risk of NMSC by approximately 78%. According to the predictions derived from our model, regular use of a SPF 4 sunscreen with an effective SPF of 2 would reduce risk of NMSC by more than 40%.

The impact of this intervention would vary with the individual's pattern of sun exposure over a lifetime and absolute level with sun exposure and innate risk. Use of sunscreens in childhood would be most effective in those individuals whose sun exposure in their early years was greatest relative to their exposure as adults.

Perhaps more important than percentage reduction in risk is the absolute reduction in risk for a group of individuals. Persons most likely to benefit from sunscreen use are those at highest risk for these tumors. The single most important determinant for risk is exposure to UVB. The determinants of exposure to UVB include the place of residence and pattern of activity. Since we relied on the federal data for solar insolation, our model takes into account latitude, altitude, and average cloud cover in calculating absolute reductions of risk.

Regular use of sunscreens in different geographical regions provides the same percentage reduction in risk. The absolute risk reduction achieved by this intervention varies greatly among areas. For example, the reduction in the number of NMSCs per 100,000 individuals would be approximately four times greater in Albuquerque, New Mexico as in Seattle, Washington. This is a result of the far higher UVB insolation and hence NMSC risk in Albuquerque. Similarly, absolute reduction of risk gained by the use of sunscreens will be greatest among individuals in a given geographic area who are genetically most prone to the development of these tumors. Among the phenotypic characteristics associated with an increased risk of NMSC are a tendency to sunburn easily and tan poorly (10). Unfortunately the very attributes that are associated with highest NMSC risk may also encourage behavior that would reduce the potential beneficial effects of the use of these agents.

VIII. FACTORS REDUCING THE BENEFITS OF SUNSCREEN USE

As a consequence of exposure to UVB, skin undergoes pigmentation and thickening of the stratum corneum. This process reduces the penetration of any subsequent UV-B to which the individual is exposed. Therefore, if an individual only sometimes uses sunscreens, the effective dose of UVB exposure reaching the basal layer of the epidermis and the dermis on days on which sunscreens were not used may be greater than had this individual not used sunscreen on previous days and had thus undergone tanning and thickening of the stratum corneum. Therefore, regular sunscreen protection throughout the seasons of the year when substantial quantities of UVB insolation occur may be needed if the full potential of these agents to prevent cancer is to be utilized.

Individuals who burn easily are at highest risk for NMSC. Before the advent of sunscreens, the duration of sun exposure was limited by the wish to avoid the sunburn that accompanied prolonged exposures. Some individuals who previously limited their exposure because of concern about sunburn may use a sunscreen as a means of extending time in the sun. In these circumstances, the use of sunscreens only slightly reduces total UV-B exposure.

In vitro studies suggest that PABA may be mutagenic. Any mutagenic effect from PABA or other constituents of sunscreens is likely to reduce the anticarcinogenic effect of these compounds.

IX. CURRENT REALITIES IN REDUCING THE RISK OF NMSC

Given the relatively greater importance of childhood sunscreen use and the relatively short period during which these compounds have been readily available and widely applied, it is unlikely that the current population at risk for NMSC could have experienced substantial reduction of risk of NMSC from the use of sunscreens even if they had regularly used these agents since they became available. At least three factors make it unlikely that the full potential benefits of using sunscreens can be realized by today's adolescents. These inhibiting factors are irregular use, using sunscreens to extend exposure, and the general population's lack of understanding about the substantial UVB exposures to which the face, neck, and arms are subject during nonrecreational periods when sunscreens are seldom used.

The earlier in life sunscreens are used, the greater is the potential for reducing the risk of NMSC. Still if, as clinical observation and our model suggest, UVB is both an initiator and promoter of cutaneous carcinogenesis, reduction in exposure to UVB by any means at any time is likely to reduce the risk of subsequent NMSC.

REFERENCES

1. Stern, R. S., Weinstein, M. C., and Baker, S. G. Risk reduction for nonmelanoma skin cancer with childhood sunscreen use. *Arch. Dermatol., 122*: 537–545 (1986).
2. Scotto, J., Fears, T. R., and Fraumeni, J. F., Jr. Skin (other than melanoma), *Incidence of nonmelanoma skin cancer in the United States*, Cancer Institute, U.S. Department of Health and Human Services (NIH) publication, Washington, D.C. (1983), pp. 82–2433.
3. Cole, C. A., Forbes, D., and Davies, R. E. An action spectrum for UV photocarcinogenesis. *Photochem. Photobiol., 43*:275–284 (1986).
4. Freeman, R. G. Data on the action spectrum for ultraviolet carcinogenesis. *JNCI, 55*:1119–1122 (1975).
5. Setlow, R. B. The wavelengths in sunlight effective in producing skin cancer: A theoretical analysis. *Proc. Natl. Acad. Sci. (USA), 64*:3363–3366 (1974).
6. Rundell, R. D. Action spectra and estimation of biologically effective UV radiation. *Physiol. Plant, 58*:360–366 (1983).

7. Fears, T. R. and Scotto, J. Estimating increases in skin cancer morbidity due to increased (sic) in ultraviolet radiation exposure. *Cancer Invest.,* *1*(2):119–126 (1983).

8. Scott, E. L. and Straf, M. L. Ultraviolet radiation as a cause of cancer, *Origins of Human Cancer, Book A, Incidence of Cancer in Humans,* Vol. 4 (H. H. Hiatt, J. D. Watson, and J. A. Winsten, eds.), The Cold Spring Laboratory, New York (1977), pp. 529–549.

9. De Gruij, F. R., Van der Meer, J. B., and Van der Leun, J. C. Dose-time dependency of tumor formation by chronic UV exposure. *Photochem. Photobiol., 37*:53–62 (1983).

10. Vitaliano, P. P. and Urbach, F. The relative importance of risk factors in nonmelanoma carcinoma. *Arch. Dermatol., 116*:454–456 (1980).

III
SUNSCREEN INGREDIENTS AND FORMULATIONS

6

Tanning Accelerators

JAMES M. WILMOTT,* MICHELE C. DUGGAN, and ALEXANDER P. ZNAIDEN *Avon Products, Inc., Suffern, New York*

I. INTRODUCTION

What is a tan? How is it formed? What does it do? Why is it there? How is it controlled?

Is tanning simply an insignificant biological phenomenon of evolutionary specialization, a primordial leftover, or a yet to be understood fractal event? Has its total purpose been missed by the researcher's eye which often looks for singularity of function, specificity of action, and black and white boundaries for definition?

Is it a sunscreen? A regulator of vitamin D synthesis? A free radical trap? A heat absorption system? A hormone? A collection and disposal system for toxic, oxidative byproducts of cellular metabolism and photodamage? A defense mechanism to protect the cell's genetic materials from ultraviolet damage?

The complete picture of the mechanisms of tanning is still unknown, but it is slowly beginning to come into focus. Scientists have elucidated the pathways of synthesis, identified cause and effect relationships, characterized the chemical composition, investigated the cells in which it is produced, and studied the consequences of unhealthy expression.

What is not well known is how to control the tanning process for aesthetic and therapeutic benefit. The following is presented to provide information on some of the agents which have demonstrated an ability to accelerate tanning and to offer suggestions which may lead to more effective materials in the future.

Current affiliation: Dow Brands, Inc., Minneapolis, Minnesota

II. THE TANNING PROCESS

It has been suggested the pigmentation response of skin may, in fact, be more than just the well-known "tanning" that occurs when one is exposed to ultraviolet light. While most people are aware of the relationship between tanning and sunlight, not many appreciate the mechanism by which this occurs. To effectively enhance tanning, such knowledge is critical and will be briefly described below.

Tanning may be simply defined as an enhancement in the production of pigment by the skin. This pigment is called melanin and it can be either black (eumelanin) or red (pheomelanin). The process by which melanin is formed is called melanogenesis. It takes place in cellular organelles known as melanosomes which are produced by epidermal melanocytes. The melanosomes contain everything that is needed for melanin production. They are transported, via melanocyticdendrites, to the epidermal keratinocytes. There are usually 36 keratinocytes associated with one melanocyte (1,2). This complex is known as the epidermal melanin unit (Fig. 1). Only when the melanin-containing melanosomes are in the keratinocytes is a tan visible.

The basic biochemical pathway of melanogenesis was elucidated by Mason and Raper, who later altered it to accommodate the contribution of all intermediates to the final product (Fig. 2). These investigators determined that the hydroxylation of the amino acid tyrosine to dopa and the oxidation of dopa to dopaquinone are under enzymatic control while the remaining steps occurred spontaneously (3). However, subsequent investigations recognized that this scheme was too simplistic because it did not account for the different types of pigments which are observed in vivo. Figure 3 demonstrates the divergence of the pathway that is due to the combination of dopaquinone with either sulfur or oxygen to form the pheomelanin or eumelanin monomer, respectively (2).

The sulfur-containing compounds of particular interest are the amino acid cysteine and the tripeptide glutathione (GSH). GSH or cysteine can be added to dopaquinone in various ways to produce four different forms of cysteinyldopa with 5-S-cysteinyldopa and 2-S-cysteinyldopa being prevalent.

The final step in this process is the polymerization of the eumelanin or pheomelanin monomers within a peptide matrix to form the characteristic black and red pigments (4,5).

III. THE ENZYME

The generally recognized key steps in melanogenesis are the conversions of tyrosine to dopa and dopa to dopaquinone, which are both catalyzed by the enzyme tyrosinase. Tyrosinase is a copper-containing protein which is usually glycosylated with neuraminic acid (also known as sialic acid), galactose, and

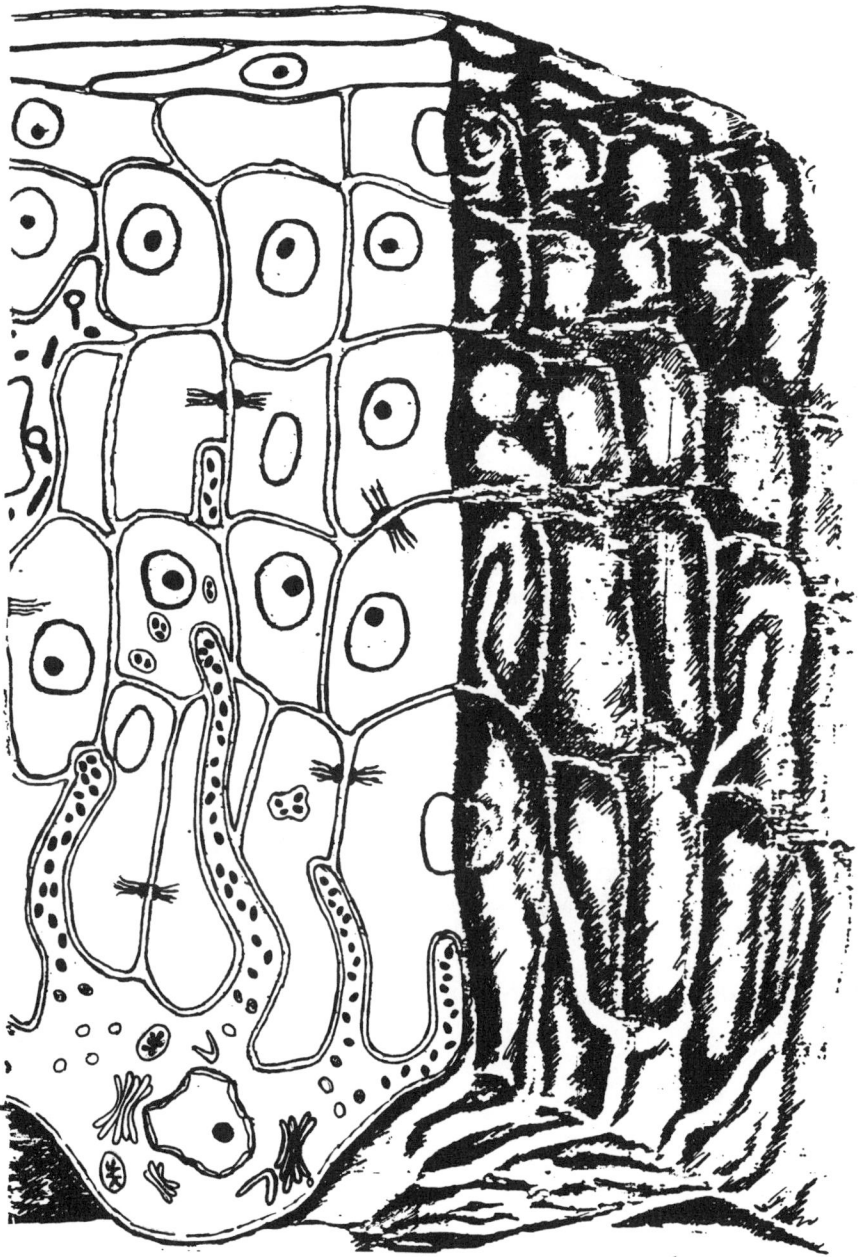

Figure 1 The epidermal melanin unit. The melanocyte (bottom) deposits pigment filled melanosomes into neighboring keratinocytes.

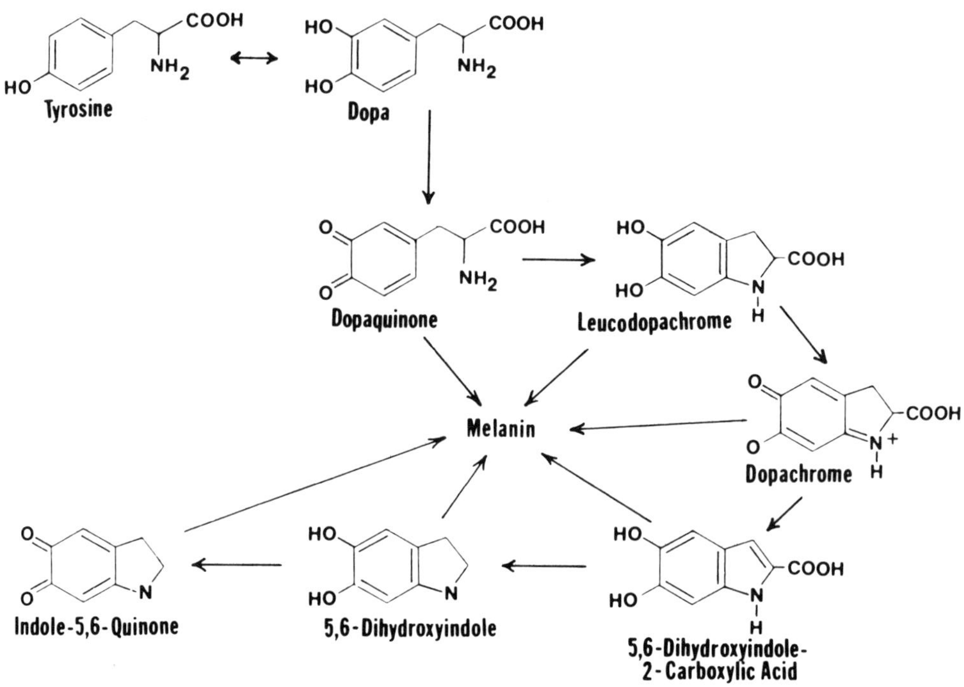

Figure 2 Mason raper pathway (from Ref. 3).

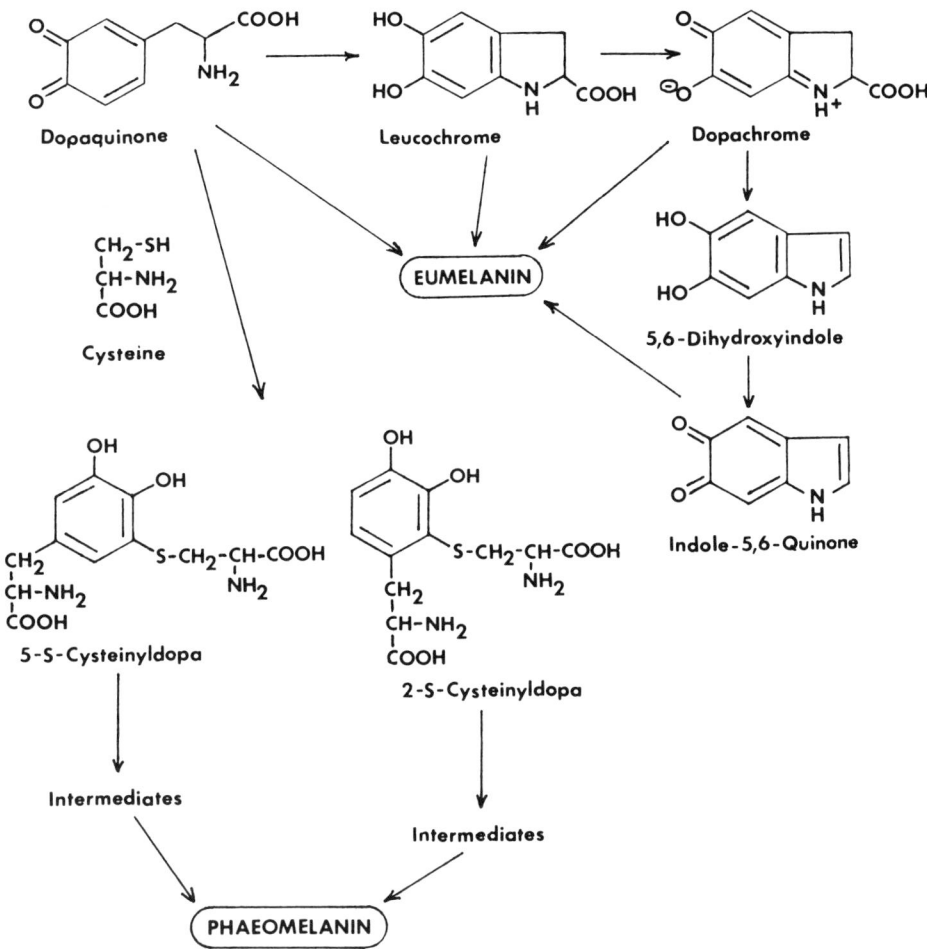

Figure 3 The biosynthetic pathway for eumelanin and pheomelanin (from Ref. 2).

possibly mannose in the active state (1,2). The protein fraction is synthesized on ribosomes which are located on the rough endoplasmic reticulum. It then migrates to a site in the Golgi apparatus via the cytoplasm or the smooth endoplasmic reticulum. Once this site is cleaved from the Golgi apparatus it is referred to as a premelanosome and exists for awhile in the cytoplasm of the melanocyte (6).

Tyrosinase, like many other enzymes, is synthesized in an inactive form termed a proenzyme which is a tetramer. McGuire et al. in their work with frog epidermis, reported that activation occurs in cytoplasmic components before the formation of premelanosomes (2). Mishima et al., in their research with B16 murine melanoma cells, confirmed that transport into the premelanosomes is necessary for melanogenic initiation (7).

In the early 1980s, Hearing et al. discovered that tyrosinase exists in three slightly different forms (isoenzymes) which have been identified as T_1, T_3, and T_4. It has been speculated that a fourth isoenzyme, T_2, existed, but this proved to be an electrophoretic artifact of T_3. T_1 and T_3 are soluble and found in the cytoplasm. They have molecular weights of 66,000 and 56,700, respectively. Together, they are responsible for only 10% of all tyrosinase activity. Both have similar enzymatic properties and are believed to be associated with an inhibitory factor. This factor has been identified by Hearing et al. as 5,6-dihydroxyindole blocking factor (IBF). As the name signifies, IBF inhibits the conversion of 5,6-dihydroxyindole to indole-5,6-quinone (2,8,9). T_4 is found bound to the melanosomal membranes, has a molecular weight of 120,000, and is responsible for approxiamtely 90% of tyrosinase activity. This high level of activity may be due to the presence of dopachrome conversion factor (DCF) and 5,6-dihydroxyindole conversion factor (ICF). The three isoenzymes also differ in carbohydrate content, T_1 and T_4 being glycosylated while T_3 is nonglycosylated (8).

Based on the research of Hearing et al. with B16 murine melanoma cells and C57Bl/6N murine hairbulbs, the researchers proposed the following pathway for tyrosinase activation. T_3 is newly synthesized by the ribosomes of the rough endoplasmic reticulum. It is then glycosylated, the sugars are added in the Golgi apparatus to form T_1. The T_1 isoenzyme is delivered to the premelanosome and is attached to the membrane to form a T_4 molecule. The authors supported this theory, in part, by incubating T_4 with the proteolytic enzyme trypsin. This cleaved the membrane fragments from T_4 and produced a molecule that was electrophoretically similar to T_1 (8).

There was much debate over whether tyrosinase was one enzyme with two functions or two enzymes, tyrosinase and dopaoxidase, each with one function. However, in recent years, researchers have identified two binding sites on the tyrosinase enzyme, one for the oxidation of dopa and the other for tyrosine (2). In fact, it has been determined that the oxidation of dopa proceeds at a faster rate than the hydroxylation of tyrosine. It has also been found that when dopa is added to a reaction mixture containing tyrosine and tyrosinase, the rate of hydroxylation is greatly increased, indicating that dopa functions as a cofactor for tyrosinase as well as a substrate (2). It is hypothesized that the increase in the reaction is due to a conformational change which enhances the efficiency of the enzyme.

While it was believed that the reactions beyond dopaquinone were spontaneous, it has been determined that tyrosinase also catalyzes the conversion of additional intermediates further along the melanogenic pathway (10). It has also been determined that these reactions are regulated by several biological factors. Pawelek's lab discovered three of these regulatory factors in mouse melanoma cells (11). DCF increases the conversion of dopachrome to 5,6 dihydroxyindole 2-carboxylate while, ICF increases the conversion of 5,6-dihydroxyindole to the

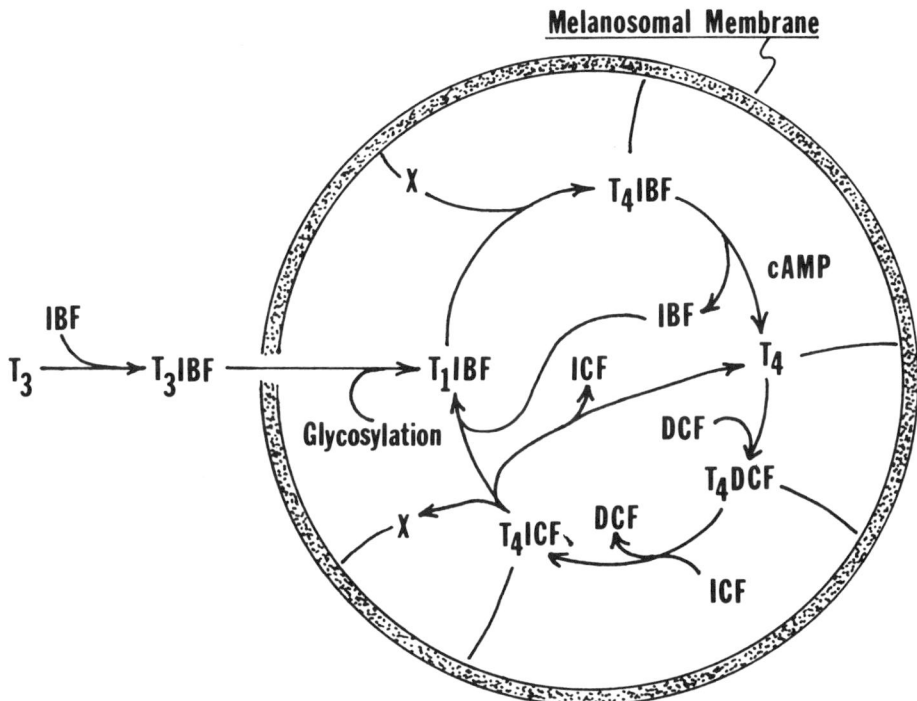

Figure 4   Proposed schematic for the activation of tyrosinase. X: membrane factor; IBF: 5,6-dihydroxyindole blocking factor; DCF: dopachrome conversion factor; ICF: 5,6-dihydroxyindole conversion factor; T_1, T_3, T_4-tyrosinase isoenzymes.

quinone and subsequently to melanin. IBF restricts melanogenesis at 5,6-di-hydroxyindole and protects cells from the cytotoxic effects of melanin precursors (12). Experiments done by Hearing et al. suggest that IBF is associated with tyrosinase isoenzymes T_1 and T_3, explaining their low level of activity (8). Both conversion factors, DCF and ICF, migrate with tyrosinase when chromatographed using both gel filtration and ion exchange columns, suggesting that the conversion factors are complexed with the isoenzymes in the pigment cells (8). This same set of experiments also suggests that DCF is associated with T_4, the most active form of tyrosinase. Figure 4 represents a hypothesis developed by Wilmott and Duggan which describes the activation of the tyrosinase isoenzymes and their relationship with the blocking and conversion factors.

From the above, one can appreciate the intricacy involved in melanogenesis. While this complexity makes the understanding of tanning more difficult, it does provide the opportunity to better comprehend how one might influence melanogenic expression. This additional knowledge might provide the cosmetic or pharmaceutical formulator with the key to develop a product that produces a tan without the need to expose the skin to high levels of damaging sunlight.

IV. SUPPORT SYSTEMS

As is the case for all enzymatic reactions, melanogenesis does not exist alone, but rather as a part of a complicated series of biochemical events. Any modification to these secondary systems can directly influence the rate and type of melanin produced. A chart identifying some of these secondary processes and their interaction with the primary melanogenic path is found in Figure 5.

A. Membrane Mediated

It is very apparent that the development of melanin is influenced by materials which bind to or complex with the membrane of the melanocyte. This "receptor" binding by an external factor produces an intracellular signal which ultimately stimulates melanogenesis.

Perhaps the most widely known material purported to be involved with melanogenesis is melanocyte-stimulating hormone (αMSH or α-Melanotropin). It is produced by the anterior portion of the pituitary gland (9). Amino acid analysis has revealed the sequence of αMSH (Fig. 6). Two peptide fragments within the αMSH have been shown to have melanogenic activity (13).

It has been fairly well established that, in melanoma cells, αMSH enhances tyrosinase activity by binding to a cell surface receptor on the melanocyte which activates the enzyme adenylate cyclase. This catalyzes the conversion of adenosine triphosphate (ATP) to cyclic adenosine monophasphate (cAMP). Calcium is needed for signal transduction, that is, the movement of the signal from the

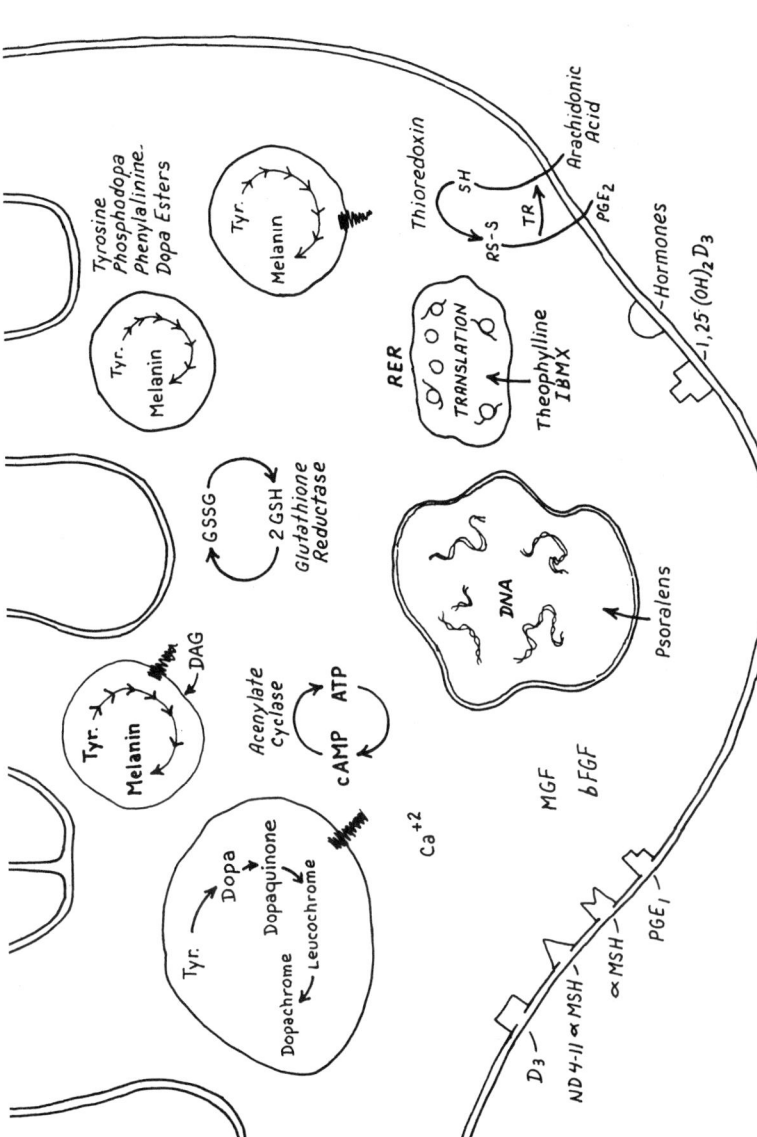

Figure 5 Support systems and agents which influence melanogenesis. DAG: diacylglycerol; GSH: glutathione; GSSG: oxidized glutathione; TR: thioredoxin reductase; RER: rough endoplasmic reticulum; IBMX: isobutylmethylxanthine; PGE_2: prostaglandin E_2; PGE_1: prostaglandin E_1; D_3: vitamin D_3; $1,25(OH)_2 D_3$: $1\alpha, 25$ dihydroxyvitamin D_3; αMSH: melanocyte stimulating hormone; MGF: melanocyte growth factor; bFGF: basic fibroblast growth factor; ATP: adenosine triphosphate; cAMP: cyclic adenosine monophosphate.

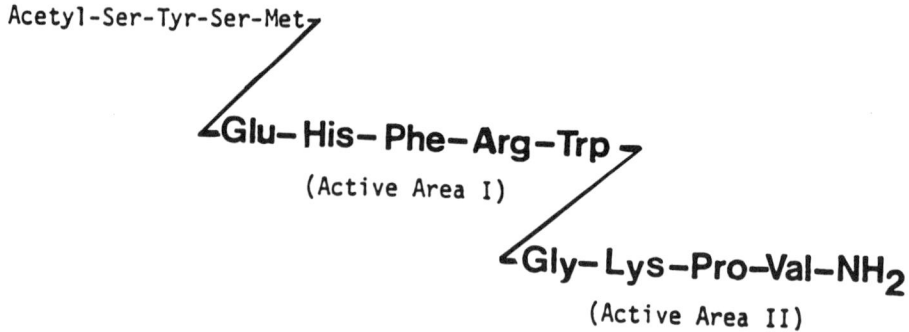

Figure 6   Amino acid sequence for MSH showing two active sites.

cell surface to the adenylate cyclase (14). The cAMP is the true activator of tyrosinase. It is thought to bind to and remove an inhibitor of tyrosinase (15). This
inhibitor may in fact be the IBF discussed by Pawelek et al., which is known to
be associated with the T_1 and T_3 isoenzymes. However, recent studies by Gilchrist have demonstrated that diacylglycerol and not cyclic AMP may serve as
the activating mechanism for nonmelanoma cells (16). cAMP was also believed
to be involved in the transfer of melanosomes into the keratinocyte as evidenced
by the increased dendricity of melanocytes in the presence of MSH (2,17).
PGE_2 has also been shown to increase melanocyte swelling and dendricity (18).
     MSH-induced activation may also occur at the genetic transcriptional or trans-
lational level through either cAMP or an alternate pathway. It has been shown
that the presence of αMSH increases the number of melanosomes. Further, Hu
et al. have demonstrated an increase in tyrosinase synthesis in mouse melanoma
cells that were treated with MSH (19).
     In addition to the two active sites in the αMSH molecule, researchers have
identified αMSH analogs which stimulate melanogenesis. The most potent analog
is Ac-[Nle 4, D-Phe 7] αMSH 4-11NH$_2$ (ND4-11 αMSH). Panasci et al. demonstrated this analog to be at least ten times more potent than αMSH in their work
with Fl variant B16 melanoma cells. They discovered that there are approximately 4500 receptors for this analog per melanoma cell (20). The investigators
theorize that once the analog complexes with a receptor, the receptor-hormone
complex is internalized into the cells followed by intracellular degradation of the
hormone (20). Hadley et al. termed ND4-11 αMSH "superpotent," having
"ultraprolonged melanogenic effects" based on their work with Cloudman S91
cells. In this model, ND4-11 αMSH was found to increase tyrosinase activity
100-fold with its melanogenic effects lasting up to 6 days after the analog was
removed from the cell culture media (21).

Other materials also affect melanogenesis through a membrane receptor mechanism. Cholera toxin, prostaglandins E_1, and possibly cholecalciferol (vitamin D_3) are believed to stimulate melanogenesis by activating adenylate cyclase (1,9).

In contrast to vitamin D_3, the hormonal form of this vitamin ($1\alpha,25$-dihydroxyvitamin D_3) increases tyrosinase activity, but not through a cyclic AMP intermediate (12). Finally, gonadal hormones such as estrogen and progesterone also enhance tyrosinase activity but their intracellular mechanisms of action have not been elucidated to date (2).

Another recently discovered membrane-bound reaction that influences pigmentation is the thioredoxin/thioredoxin reductase system. Thioredoxin is a flavoprotein present in the plasma membrane of both the melanocyte and keratinocyte. It is involved in the reduction of oxygen free radicals. It requires intracellular NADPH to accomplish the reduction of superoxide anion radicals. Oxidized thioredoxin in the presence of tyrosinase, enhances the conversion of tyrosine to melanin. Reduced thioredoxin decreases the conversion of tyrosine to DOPA even in the presence of tyrosinase (22). This finding is particularly significant since many of the mediators for reactions which cause enhanced pigmentation occur via a free radical mechanism. In fact, many of the processes involved in the inflammation processes generate free radicals of arachidonic acid (e.g., certain prostaglandins and leukotrienes). This process may represent the mechanism by which chronic irritation and sunlight achieve their melanogenic effect.

B. Intracellular Mechanisms

Within the cell, a number of peripheral events occur which influence the rate and manifestation of melanogenesis. Of particular importance is the role of deoxyribonucleic acid (DNA).

DNA is at the core of all cellular activity because all molecules produced by cells are ultimately under DNA control. In melanogenesis, factors which direct the expression of DNA may enhance (or inhibit) either the availability of key melanogenic components or the proliferation of the melanocyte itself. In the former, either transcriptional or translational properties may be influenced. In the latter, the synthesis of DNA itself is enhanced resulting in increased mitotic activity.

Materials which are theorized to promote tanning by their effect on DNA are psoralens. In 1974, Carter et al. demonstrated in vitro stimulation of tyrosinase activity by trimethyl psoralen (TMP) and by 8-methoxypsoralen (8-MOP) in conjunction with UVA exposure (23). In 1983, Borkovic et al., in their work with mouse melanoma cells, discovered that 8-MOP requires UVA exposure while TMP functions in the absence of ultraviolet light (24). It has been purported that the different pigmentary effects of TMP and 8-MOP, along with different binding sites on the nuclear DNA, support the hypothesis of DNA level regulation (23).

Other materials such as melanocyte growth factor and basic fibroblast growth factor accelerate the growth cycle of the melanocyte in culture. This enhances the mitogenic activity of the cells (25).

Finally, many other intracellular biochemical reactions are required to support the melanogenic process. In fact, proper homeostasis is required for optimum cell function. Any modification of those systems (e.g., the selective stimulation or inhibition of a key enzyme such as glutathione reductase) might have profound consequences on the development of melanin.

Evidence for the influential effect of the support systems in the development of pigmentation is found in the myriad chemicals and physiological disorders which result in hyperpigmentation (17,26,27). Most of these conditions act at a different site on or within the melanocyte (Table 1). This diversity of action has recently given rise to speculation that melanogenesis is much more than the development of color due to exposure of the skin to UV radiation. Rather, the conversion of tyrosine to melanin may be the mechanism for the ultimate removal of oxidative damage from the skin.

V. TANNING ACCELERATORS

Since the close of World War II, the possession of a tan has been associated with available leisure time and, social success. The cosmetic value of pigmentation has generated a proliferation of consumer products claiming to enhance or "accelerate" the tanning process. The early 1980s ushered in the era of tan accelerators which successfully created a niche in the sun products category. Today more than 15 product lines are marketed for the purpose of enhanced tanning. The rapid proliferation of tanning accelerators confirms the consumer desire for pro-pigmenting products. However, there is also a pharmacological need to develop these products to improve the outward appearance of pigmentary disorders, such as melasma, listed in Table 1 (27).

As discussed above, pigmentation is a complex series of biochemical reactions which can be affected by a wide variety of materials and conditions. A broader understanding of the many mechanisms involved will help formulators to identify materials which can safely modify the tanning process.

A. Direct Manipulation of the Melanogenic Path

Most of the currently marketed tanning accelerators contain tyrosine, tyrosine derivatives, tyrosine/riboflavin (or ATP) complexes, and/or amino acid blends. Tyrosine is used to increase the substrate available for tyrosinase (28); however, this approach may have some limitations because:

Table 1 Factors Involved with Promoting Pigmentation

Source	Melanocytotic (increase in number of melanocytes)	Melanotic (increase in melanin)
Heritable or developmental	Lentigines	Cafe au lait macule
	Moynahan's syndrome	Neurofibromatosis
	Centrofacial neurodysraphic lentiginosis	Albright's syndrome
	Peutz-Jegher syndrome	Silver Russel syndrome
	PUVA	Westerhof syndrome
	Soto syndrome	Watson syndrome
		Bloom syndrome
		Gastrocutaneous syndrome
		Becker's melanosis
		Nevus spilus
		Ephelides (freckles)
		Name/Lamb syndrome
		Ichthyosis nigricans
		Neurocutaneous melanosis
		Familial periorbital hyperpigmentation
		Familial progressive hyperpigmentation
		Dowling Degos disease
		Dyskeratosis congenita
		Fanconi's syndrome
		Human chimaera
		Acropigmentation of Dotti
		Reticulate acropigmentation of Kitamura
		Dermatopathia pigmentosa reticularis
		Poems syndrome
		Carbon baby syndrome

Table 1 (Continued)

Source	Melanocytotic (increase in number of melanocytes)	Melanotic (increase in melanin)
Metabolic		Porphyria cutanea tarda Hemochromatosis Hepholenticular degeneration Gaucher's disease Niemann-Pick disease
Endocrine		Melasma ACTH- and MSH-producing tumors Exogenous ACTH therapy Pregnancy Addison's disease Estrogen therapy
Chemical and drug		Arsenicals Busulfan Photochemical agents (psoralens, tar) Berlock dermatosis 5-Fluorouracil, systemic Cyclophosphamide Nitrogen mustard, topical Bleomycin

Physical	Lentigo, solar Ultraviolet radiation (tanning)	Ultraviolet radiation (suntanning) Thermal radiation Alpha, beta, gamma ionizing radiation Trauma (e.g., chronic pruritus)
Inflammation and infection		Postinflammatory melanosis (exanthems, drug eruptions) Lichen planus Lupus erythematosus, discoid Lichen simplex chronicus Atopic dermatitis Psoriasis Tinea versicolor
Neoplastic		Melanoma Mastocytosis Acanthosis nigricans with adenocarcinoma and lymphoma
Miscellaneous	Lentigines, eruptive Lentigo, senile	Scleroderma, systemic Chronic hepatic insufficiency Whipple's syndrome Cronkhite-Canada syndrome

Source: From Ref. 27.

1. Tyrosine may not penetrate the skin
2. Tyrosine has low water solubility, therefore, the amount in the skin may not be greatly increased
3. The concentration of tyrosine in the skin may already be at the maximum level for what the enzyme can handle

Any of these factors could jeopardize the efficacy of the tanning accelerator (29).

A glucose ester of tyrosine, glucose tyrosinate, has been developed to overcome the low water solubility of tyrosine, thereby permitting greater amounts of the amino acid to be present in the skin. Tyrosine was also complexed with riboflavin or ATP in order to accelerate its oxidation. Work by Okun et al. also demonstrated that the enzyme peroxidase can rapidly hydroxylate tyrosine to dopa in melanoma cells (30). Finally, amino acid blends are added to provide precursors of tyrosine in addition to increasing diffusability in the skin (31). While a rationale for the use of these materials can be developed, there are questions concerning the magnitude of the effect that can be delivered.

Collaborative work done by Yale University and Plough indicates that phosphodopa and its derivatives increase melanogeneses. This may be accomplished by increasing the amount of substrate/cofactor for the dopaoxidase function of tyrosinase (32). This approach is further supported by Yu and Van Scott, who patented the use of esters of dopa to enhance pigmentation in hair and skin (33).

B. Modification of the Melanogenic Support Systems

Release of Tyrosinase Inhibition

Hadley's work with vertebrate pigment cells indicates that tyrosinase inhibition can be released by increasing the level of cyclic AMP (cAMP), which is thought to bind to and remove an inhibitor of tyrosinase (15). This can be accomplished by the direct introduction of cAMP and derivatives of cAMP (e.g., dibutyryl cAMP) or by stimulating the activity of the enzyme adenylate cyclase. The latter can be achieved by the addition of αMSH, cholera toxin, prostaglandin E_1, or vitamin D_3, all of which are believed to bind membrane-bound receptors (1,9). Of particular interest is the dramatic stimulatory effect that can be achieved through a series of MSH analogs developed by Hadley. The most potent analog being the Ac-[Nle-4, D-Phe-7] αMSH 4-11-NH2 (ND 4-11 αMSH).

An intriguing possibility for enhanced melanogenesis is the use of diacyl glycerol (DAG). Of particular interest is 1,2-dicapryloylglycerol. It is speculated that the release of tyrosinase inhibitors in a normal nonmalignant melanocyte may occur via DAG and not through cAMP (16). An investigation of the promoting effect of various acyl group appears warranted.

DNA Regulation

As discussed previously, by affecting the genetic expression of the melanocyte (DNA), one can alter melanogenesis. Psoralens are believed to function this way by binding to sites on the DNA molecule. Currently, the well-known psoralens (TMP and 8-MOP) are not available for use in cosmetic products due to safety concerns. However, efficacious psoralen-like materials possessing lower toxicity may be possible. The resurgence in the investigation of natural products may help identify such materials.

Another way to increase melanogenesis through use of the genetic system is to increase the amount of tyrosinase present in the melanosome. Hu et al. demonstrated that theophylline may directly increase the rate of tyrosinase synthesis (19). Since theophylline has demonstrated efficacy in this area, it may also be possible for other xanthine base derivatives such as caffeine, theobromine, and isobutyl methylxanthine (IBMX) to have a similar effect.

Finally, a logical way to enhance melanogenesis is to increase the number of melanocytes. While work in this area is relatively new, recent experiments have successfully identified several key materials required for the proliferation of melanocytes in vitro. Cell culture studies conducted by Gilchrist et al. have shown that materials such as melanocyte growth factor, basic fibroblast growth factor, prostaglandin E_2, and other serum factors are needed for promoting cell growth (25). Other agents, such as choleratoxin, have also been employed to enhance the proliferation of melanocytes in culture.

While the efficacy of such materials appears inviting, the short-term use of them is remote. However, as research continues in this area there is every hope that the judicious application of a carefully selected agent might enhance cell proliferation without the oncological consequences that might accompany the improper use of mitogens.

Utilization of Conversion Factors

An interesting possibility to control the development of pigment may be found by enhancing the apparent effect of the conversion factors DCF and ICF. It is possible that DCF and ICF function by removing IBF-related inhibition while structurally modifying the conformation of the enzyme to permit a more rapid conversion to 5,6 dihydroxyindole-2-carboxylic acid and indole 5,6-quinone, respectively. If this is the case, then increasing the amount of the conversion factors would result in increased tyrosinase activity. Unfortunately, neither the conversion factors nor their mechanisms of action are well understood. However, greater knowledge in this area might provide a unique opportunity to enhance pigmentation.

Miscellaneous

Several membrane-mediated events produce a propigmentary effect without the involvement of cAMP. $1\alpha,25$ dihydroxyvitamin D_3 and certain steroidal hormones (e.g., estrogen) have been shown to have efficacy. These findings suggest that analogs of these agents might selectively promote tanning without the obvious toxicological consequences associated with the use of high levels of the parent compound.

Finally, the efforts of Woods et al. with their discovery of the role of the thioredoxin/thioredoxin reductase system in the release and inhibition of tyrosinase may offer unique opportunities to promote pigmentation. Materials which could selectively oxidize thioredoxin or inhibit the reductase enzyme would increase the level of available tyrosinase.

VI. CONCLUSION

Scientists appear to be on the verge of unraveling the total role of the melanocyte and the melanogenic process. Several have demonstrated that there is a close interaction between the melanocyte, the keratinocyte and the Langerhans cell in the epidermis. Further, communication from the dermal fibroblast as well as mediators circulating in the blood have shown the ubiquitous involvement of melanogenesis in maintaining the health of the body. These interactions confirm that "tanning" is a dynamic process, one which will require the investigator to have a broad perspective in order to moderate it safely.

REFERENCES

1. Fitzpatrick, T. B., Eisen, A. Z., Wolfe, K., Freedman, I. M., and Austen, K. F. *Dermatology in General Medicine*, 2nd Ed. McGraw-Hill, New York (1979).
2. McGuire, J., Newman, D., and Barisas, G. Tyrosinase-protyrosinase system in frog epidermis, *Yale J. Biol. Med., 46* (5):572-582 (1973).
3. Prota, G. Recent advances in the chemistry of melanogenesis in mammals. *J. Invest. Dermatol., 75* (1):122-127 (1980).
4. Prota, G. Some new aspects of eumelanin chemistry, *Advances in Pigment Cell Research* (J. T. Bagnara, ed.), Alan R. Liss, New York (1988), pp. 116-118.
5. Jimbrow, K., Yamana, K., Akutsu, Y., and Maeda, K. Nature and biosynthesis of structural matrix protein in melanosomes: Melanosomal structural protein as differentiation antigen for neoplastic melanocytes, *Advances in Pigment Cell Research* (J. T. Bagnara, ed.), Alan R. Liss, New York (1988), pp. 169-172.

6. Hearing, V. J. and Jimenez, M. Mammalian tyrosinase—the critical regulatory control point in melanocyte pigmentation. *Int. J. Biochem., 19*(12): 1141-1147 (1987).

7. Mishima, Y. and Imokawa, G. Selective aberration and pigment loss in melanosomes of malignant melanoma cells in vitro by glycosylation inhibitors: Premalanosomes as glycoprotein. *J. Invest. Dermatol., 81*(2): 106-114 (1983).

8. Hearing, V. J., Korner, A. M., and Pawelek, J. M. New regulators of melanogenesis are associated with purified tyrosinase isoenzymes. *J. Invest. Dermatol., 79*(10):16-18 (1982).

9. Goldsmith, L. A. (Ed.). *Biochemistry and Physiology of the Skin*, Oxford University Press, New York (1983).

10. Korner, A. and Pawelek, J. Mammalian tyrosinase catalyses three reactions in the biosynthesis of melanin. *Science, 217*(4565):1163-1165 (1982).

11. Pawelek, J., Korner, A., Bergstrom, A., and Bologna, J. New regulators of melanin biosynthesis and the autodestruction of melanoma cells. *Nature, 286*:617-619 (1980).

12. Hosoi, J., Abe, E., Suba, T., and Kuroki, T. Regulation of melanin synthesis of B-16 mouse melanoma cells by 1-alpha 25 dihydroxyvitamin D-3 and retinoic-acid. *Cancer Res., 45*(4):1474-1478 (1985).

13. Eberle, A. M. Studies on melanotropin (MSH) receptors of melanophores and melanoma cells. *Biochem. Soc. Trans., 9*(1):37-39 (1981).

14. Lucas, A. M., Thody, A. J., and Shuster, S. The role of calcium in MSH stimulated melanosome dispersion. *Peptides, 8*(6):955-960 (1987).

15. Hadley, M. E., Heward, C. B., Hruby, V. J., Sawyer, T. K., and Young, Y. C. S. Hormone receptors and vertebrate pigment cells. *Yale J. Biol. Med., 53*:385-448 (1980).

16. Gilchrist, B. Tufts University, Boston, MA, personal communication (1988).

17. Nordlund, J. J., Sober, A. J., and Hansen, T. W. Periodic synopsis on pigmentation. *J. Am. Acad. Dermatol., 12*(2):359-363 (1985).

18. Tomita, Y., Iwamoto, M., Masuda, T., and Tagami, H. Stimulatory effect of prostaglanelin E-2 on the configuration of normal human melanocytes in vitro. *J. Invest. Dermatol., 89*(3):299-301 (1987).

19. Hu, F., Mah, K., and Teramure, D. J. Electron microscopic and cytochemical observations of theophylline and melanocyte-stimulating hormone effects on melanoma cells in culture. *Cancer Res., 42*:2786-2791 (1982).

20. Panasci, L. C., McQuillan, A., and Kaufman, M. Biological activity, binding, and metabolic fate of Ac-[Nle4, D-Phe7] alpha-MSH4-11NH$_2$, with the Fl variant of B16 melanoma cells. *J. Cell Physiol., 132*(1):97-103 (1987).

21. Hadley, M. E., Abdel Malek, A. Z., Marivan, M. M., Kreutzfeld, K. L., and Hruby, V. J. [Nle4, D-Phe 7]-alpha-MSH: A superpotent melanotropin that irreversibly activates melanoma tyrosinase. *Endocr. Res., 11*(3-4):157-70 (1985).

22. Schalleuter, K. U., Pittelkow, M. R., and Wood, J. M. Free radical reduction by thioredoxin reductase at the surface of normal and vitiliginous human keratinocytes. *J. Invest. Dermatol., 87*:728-732 (1986).

23. Carter, D. M., Wolff, K., and Schnedl, W. 8-Methoxypsoralen and UVA promote sister chromatid exchanges. *J. Invest. Dermatol., 67*(4):548–551 (1976).
24. Borkovic, S. P., Alper, J. C., and McDonald, C. J. Stimulation of pigmentation in melanoma cells by trimethyl psoralen in the absence of UV irradiation. *Br. J. Dermatol., 108*(5):525–532 (1983).
25. Gilchrist, B. Tufts University, Boston, MA, personal communication (1987).
26. Ortonne, J. P. Chemical and drug induced hypermelanoses, *Advances in Pigment Cell Research* (J. T. Bognara, ed.), Alan R. Liss, New York (1988), pp. 116–118.
27. Fitzpatrick, T. B., Eisen, A. Z., Wolfe, K., Freedberg, I. M., and Austen, K. F. *Dermatology in General Medicine*, Third Ed., McGraw-Hill, New York (1987), pp. 838–876.
28. Pawelek, J., Bolognia, J., McLane, J., Murray, M., Osber, M., and Slominski, A. A possible role for melanin precursors in regulating both pigmentation and proliferation of melanocytes, *Advances in Pigment Cell Research* (J. T. Bagnara, ed.), Alan R. Liss, New York (1988), pp. 143–154.
29. Agin, P. P., Wilson, D. K., Shorter, G. G., and Sayre, R. M. Tyrosine does not enhance tanning. *Bioscience 33*(8):516–517 (1983).
30. Okun, M., Edelstein, L., Or, N., Hamada, G., Donnellan, B., and Burnett, J. Oxidation of tyrosine and dopa to melanin by mammalian peroxidase: The possible role of peroxidase in melanin and catecholamine synthesis in vivo, *Pigmentation: Its Genesis and Biological Control* (V. Riley, ed.), Appleton-Century-Crofts, New York (1972).
31. Pauly, M., European patent 0,010,483 (1980).
32. Plough, Inc., AU 8,426,243 (1984).
33. Yu, R. J. and Van Scott, E. J., U.S. patent 4,021,538 (1977).

7
5-Methoxypsoralen-Containing Sunscreens

ANTONY R. YOUNG *United Medical and Dental Schools of Guy's and St. Thomas's Hospitals, University of London, London, England*

I. INTRODUCTION

A. Conventional Sunscreens

The purpose of most sunscreen preparations is to absorb solar ultraviolet radiation and prevent skin damage. In general, the active molecules absorb primarily in the UVB (290–315 nm) part of the solar spectrum (1). Efficacy of these preparations is assessed by their sun protection factors (SPFs) (2). More recently there has been an interest in UVA- (315–400 nm) absorbing sunscreens, especially in UVA-sensitive individuals (3,4), but the importance of such preparations on normal skin has yet to be fully determined.

It is now widely recognized that sunscreen use, especially in the more sun-sensitive skin types I and II, is important in preventing the acute effects of solar exposure, viz erythema (2), and animal data suggest an important role in preventing or delaying established long-term effects of solar radiation such as skin cancer (5) and photoageing (6,7). Increasingly, it is being advocated that sunscreens be used not just on the beach or during outdoor leisure activities but also while outdoors generally (8,9), especially in sunny climates.

One of the, probably many, areas of resistance of sunscreen use is the reduction of tanning that is associated with good sunscreen photoprotection, especially in people who do not tan readily. It is obvious that a tan is still a highly valued cosmetic and social asset despite much publicized dermatological opinion against excessive solar exposure and UVA sunbed use.

The application of an effective sunscreen will enable the user to (i) spend longer in the sun in order to obtain a given multiple of a minimal erythema dose

(MED) or (ii) prevent or reduce erythema if the amount of time spent in the sun is similar to that spent without the sunscreen. The former option may actually increase the long-term risks of solar exposure (8), especially as the use of UVB sunscreens (to prolong solar exposure time) will result in increased exposure to solar UVA. It has been demonstrated experimentally that, on an MED equivalent basis, UVA and UVB show similar carcinogenic potential (10).

B.   5-Methoxypsoralen-Containing Sunscreens

About 15 years ago, UVB sunscreen preparations which contained 5-methoxy-psoralen (5-MOP) appeared on the European market. 5-MOP is a natural furo-coumarin present at about 3000–3600 ppm in the fragrant oil extracted from the rind of the bergamot fruit (Citrus bergamia) (11,12). The rationale behind the addition of 5-MOP to conventional sunscreens is that UVB erythema (and tanning) are inhibited by the sunscreens but 5-MOP, at a final concentration of 10–50 ppm, in bergamot oil enhances melanogenesis in the presence of solar UVA (13). 5-MOP has long been recognized as the pigmentary agent in berloque dermatitis (14). The characteristics of this disorder were "pendant"-like areas of hyperpigmentation on sun-exposed sites of the neck after application of eau de cologne or other bergamot oil-containing perfumes. Berloque dermatitis is rarely seen nowadays, probably because of a reduction in the concentration of 5-MOP in perfume products. Current recommended maximum level of 5-MOP in final fragrance products is 15 ppm (International Fragrance Association, 1978).

II.   PHOTOMUTAGENICITY AND PHOTOCARCINOGENICITY OF PSORALENS

Much of the photochemical/photobiological research on the psoralens has been concentrated on an isomer of 5-MOP, viz, 8-methoxypsoralen (8-MOP) which is widely used in conjunction with UVA radiation (PUVA) in the treatment of psoriasis (15). 8-MOP and 5-MOP form unstable complexes with DNA in the dark (16,17), but in the presence of UVA, both psoralens photobind to DNA (18,19). Such photobinding, which is chemically stable, is associated with the many of the photobiological effects of these compounds. For example, 8-MOP and 5-MOP show potent mutagenicity, in bacterial, yeast, and mammalian systems, in the presence of UVA radiation (20,21). In general, 8-MOP and 5-MOP show similar photobiological properties but often with quantitative differences. In the absence of UVA, the psoralens generally show no biological activity, but frameshift mutations have been observed in bacteria with 5-MOP and other psoralens (21).

It has long been established that 8-MOP is a photocarcinogen in mouse skin (22,23), but the significance of psoralens in human skin carcinogenesis has not been unequivocally established. An extensive epidemiological study of psoriatic patients on 8-MOP photochemotherapy in the United States has provided convincing evidence that PUVA is a carcinogen (24). An important aspect of this study was the relationship between PUVA dose and skin cancer. However, a long-term study published by a group of European investigators did not support the American observations that PUVA was a complete carcinogen, but indicated that it was a promoting agent (25). The reasons for the different conclusions are not established but possible explanations have been discussed by Gibbs et al. (26).

Few data on human skin 5-MOP photocarcinogenicity are available. 5-MOP has been proposed as a better agent than 8-MOP in PUVA (27), but there have been no long-term followup studies in patients. An epidemiological study on workers in the bergamot oil production industry (28) did not find any evidence of an increased incidence of skin cancer in comparison with a control group. However, an IARC working group noted some limitations in this study (29).

Studies by Zajdela and Bisagni (30) and Young et al. (31) have clearly shown 5-MOP to be a skin photocarcinogen in mice after prolonged exposure. This has been recognized by an IARC working group (29). Comparative data from one study (30) indicated that 8-MOP was more potent than 5-MOP but data from the study of Young et al. (31) indicated similar photocarcinogenic potential. The experimental photocarcinogenicity of 5-MOP is not surprising given the potent mutagenicity of this molecule, in a variety of systems, in the presence of UVA (20,21,32). In addition, 5-MOP, as with 8-MOP, induces epidermal ornithine decarboxylase (ODC) activity (33). Induction of ODC activity has been associated with tumor promotion in chemical carcinogenesis of the skin (34,35).

The photocarcinogenicity data described in the above studies were derived from 5-MOP (100–300 ppm) in oily or acetone vehicles without UVB sunscreens in albino mice. Zajdela and Bisagni (30) used a UVA source, but Young et al. (31) used solar-simulating radiation (SSR) which is more relevant to natural solar exposure. Cartwright and Walter (36) published data which indicated that a commercially available oil-based 5-MOP sunscreen preparation enhanced photo-tumorigenesis in mouse skin. It has also been reported that a commercially available 5-MOP-containing sunscreen induced ODC activity in mouse skin exposed to UVB + UVA (37). Theoretically, such data are more relevant to human use but these experiments lacked vehicle (with and without sunscreen) controls and it has been demonstrated that an oily vehicle enhances photocarcinogenesis (31, 38). A more recent study, with the necessary controls, by Young et al. (39) has shown that low concentration UVB sunscreens (Parsol MCX; 2-ethylyhexyl 4'-methoxycinnamate with Ultracyd; 1,7,7-tri-methyl-3-benzylidene-bicyclo-[2.2.1]-2-heptanone) can have very marked inhibitory effects on 5-MOP-enhanced photocarcinogenesis. Animals were irradiated daily with SSR for about 45 weeks. Thereafter, half the animals were sacrificed and half were followed up without irradiation for 15 weeks. Comprehensive statistical analysis of the data showed that although 5-MOP was a photocarcinogen in the absence of UVB sunscreens, the addition of the sunscreens completely inhibited any enhancement by 5-MOP during the irradiation period of 45 weeks. Thus the groups treated with 5-MOP plus sunscreen were not significantly different from the groups treated with sunscreens alone. If the analyses were carried out for the total period (i.e., irradiation and follow-up), the majority of the statistical evaluations showed no difference between the 5-MOP plus sunscreen group and sunscreen only group, but a few analyses did indicate some evidence of increased risk in the 5-MOP groups. The main conclusions from these data were that the risks from the addition of 5-MOP to sunscreens were very much lower than had been previously feared from earlier data.

The marked protective effect of Parsol MCX alone against 5-MOP photo-tumorigenesis was confirmed in another study (40) with Skh 1 hairless albino mice treated with preparations in a lotion base. However, in this study 5-MOP plus sunscreen was significantly more phototumorigenic than sunscreen alone after 60 weeks of SSR exposure. These studies also compared Skh 1 mice with hairless pigmented mice of the same strain (Skh 2). Both types of mouse showed similar susceptibility to tumors, but it must be noted that epidermal melano-genesis did not occur in the dorsal skin of the Skh 2 mice although this mouse shows a good pigmentation response in ear epidermis (41).

III. POSSIBLE MECHANISMS OF SUNSCREEN PROTECTION WITH 5-MOP

It is well known that psoralens are activated by UVA. Radiation sources used in PUVA usually have an emission peak at about 365 nm and UVA sunscreens have been shown to inhibit 5-MOP-induced erythema in the guinea pig (42). Thus, initially, it may seem surprising that UVB sunscreens should inhibit 5-MOP phototumorigenesis. It should not be forgotten that psoralen absorption spectra generally have maxima in the region of 300 nm. The majority of psoralen action spectrum studies in biological systems have been done with 8-MOP. These studies show that the waveband 320–340 nm is the most important for end-points such as erythema (43), sunburn cell formation (44), inhibition of epidermal DNA synthesis (45), inhibition of mitogen-induced DNA synthesis in lymphocytes (46), and inhibition of growth in yeast (47). Recently, it has been shown by Young et al. that the 320–340 nm waveband is also the most significant in 8-MOP photocarcinogenesis (48). 5-MOP action spectra data are limited, but such that are available suggest that they are similar to 8-MOP (49,50). The only psoralen action spectrum for pigmentation appears to be with 4,5'-8-trimethylpsoralen in the guinea pig in which a maximal plateau was seen at 330–350 nm (50).

UVB sunscreens, such as Parsol MCX (2-ethylhexyl 4′-methoxycinnamate), show significant absorbance in the 320–335 nm region (39). Thus it seems reasonable to suppose that the inhibition of photocarcinogenesis by Parsol MCX is due to optical filtering of relevant wavelengths of the action spectrum. However, Parsol MXC has been shown to quench the 5-MOP triplet state (51) which may be important in psoralen/DNA photobinding (52). Thus protection may also be occurring at a more fundamental photophysical level.

IV. PHOTOCHEMOPROTECTION

Much of the data on the tanning efficacy of psoralens, especially 8-MOP, have been anecdotal but efficacy has been confirmed (53) and PUVA is used as a means of treating vitiligo (54). One laboratory study indicated that 5-MOP-containing sunscreens did not enhance pigmentation (55), but it is possible that subjects were not observed for a long enough period. Field studies have provided evidence that 5-MOP-containing sunscreens do enhance tanning (56,57). Such preparations do enhance epidermal melanogenesis in the ear of the pigmented Skh 2 mouse (41), but not in dorsal skin (40).

Photochemoprotection has been demonstrated with 8-MOP in normal subjects using such endpoints as prevention of erythema (58,59), DNA damage, and sunburn cell formation (60). The underlying design of such experiments was to induce pigmentation with 8-MOP and UVR and then, at a later stage, challenge the tanned site with UVR alone and make comparisons with a non-8-MOP tanned site which had received a similar challenge. A PUVA tan is also used prophylactically in patients with sun-sensitive skins (3,61).

Until recently, evidence of photochemoprotection with 5-MOP has not been available. Sambuco et al. (62) showed that, under some conditions, a 5-MOP-containing sunscreen induced a tan that inhibited SSR-induced sunburn cell formation in the skin of the miniature pig. Sunburn cells are thought to be a consequence of keratinocyte DNA damage (63). Direct evidence of 5-MOP-induced protection against SSR-induced DNA damage in human keratinocytes in vivo has been shown by Young et al. (64) and Potten et al. (65). In these studies, previously untanned sites of the buttocks of skin type II subjects were tanned with sunscreens, with and without 5-MOP, and SSR alone. This was done by exposing the sites to 0.7 MED for 10 consecutive weekdays. One week after the final tanning treatment, the sites were challenged with 2 MED (determined on untanned skin) SSR. Biopsies were taken and assessed for unscheduled DNA synthesis (UDS) as a marker of repair of SSR-induced DNA damage. UDS comparisons of pretreated sites were made with a site that was challenged, but not previously tanned. The data show that sites treated with sunscreen alone resulted in minimal tanning and afforded no protection from DNA damage. Protection from sites treated with sunscreen plus 5-MOP was 5-MOP dose dependent and ranged

Table 1 Unscheduled DNA Synthesis (UDS), Tanning, and Skin Thickness in 4 Skin Type II Volunteers

Treatment[a]/challenge[b]	UDS		Melanin histology[e]	Visual[f]	Skin thickening	
	counts[c]	%[d]			counts[f]	%[h]
None/none	0.6	0.08	1.0	0	14.7	95
None/SSR	7.6	100	1.7	0	15.5	100
SSR/SSR	6.4	84	5.0	3.5	27.5	177
S+SSR/SSR	7.4	97	2.0	1.0	18.0	116
S+15 ppm 5-MOP+SSR/SSR	4.2	55	4.8	3.5	20.0	129
S+30 ppm 5-MOP+SSR/SSR	2.7	36	5.5	4.5	25.1	162
S+45 ppm 5-MOP+SSR/SSR	2.5	33	5.6	4.5	23.5	152

[a]10 consecutive weekdays; 0.7 MED SSR.
[b]2 MED SSR 1 week after last tanning treatment.
[c]Mean no grains/basal cell nucleus.
[d]As above, but expressed as %age of no treatment/SSR challenge count.
[e]Graded scoring system 0-6.
[f]Graded scoring system 0-5.
[g]No cell layers in stratum corneum.
[h]As above, but expressed as %age of no treatment/SSR challenge count.
Abbreviations: S, sunscreens; 2% Parsol MCX + 1% Eusolex 6300; SSR, solar-simulated radiation.
Data modified from Ref. 64.

from about 40 to 60%. Surprisingly, mean data (12 individuals; 3 experiments) from sites tanned with SSR alone did not show protection (65), although some protection was apparent in some individuals. The results from one experiment with skin type II volunteers are summarized in Table 1. Preliminary unpublished experiments by Potten and Young indicate a similar pattern of photoprotection in skin type I despite the poor tans observed in these subjects. A tan induced by SSR alone afforded no protection from sunburn cell damage in pig skin (62). In a separate human experiment, it was shown that a 5-MOP-containing sunscreen tan afforded partial protection for up to three months. When such a tan (at about 3 months) was re-exposed to SSR alone, protection was better than an SSR alone tan re-exposed to SSR alone under the same conditions (65).

V. RISK/BENEFIT ANALYSIS

The data on 5-MOP photomutagenicity and photocarcinogenicity have prompted widespread concern and discussion about the use of 5-MOP in sunscreens (2,13, 21,29,30,66-68). This concern is valid given that 5-MOP and 8-MOP show similar photocarcinogenic potential in mice (31) and that there is good evidence that 8-MOP is photocarcinogenic in human skin (24).

Although the animal phototumorigenesis studies with 5-MOP and sunscreens (39,40) show differences in the degree of protection afforded by the sunscreen(s) from 5-MOP-enhanced phototumorigenesis, it is evident that UVB sunscreens are highly effective in this respect. Thus the photocarcinogenic risk associated with the use of 5-MOP in sunscreens must be much lower than previously feared from photomutagenicity and photocarcinogenicity data without sunscreens. However, this risk has not been eliminated.

It should also be noted that the dorsal epidermis of mice in the 5-MOP photo-carcinogenicity studies was incapable of tanning and was treated 5 days/week for about half the life span of a mouse, but that human use of 5-MOP-containing sunscreens is likely to be intermittent. Despite the protective effects of the UVB filter and the likely differences in exposure patterns of laboratory mice and humans, it is apparent that the experimental carcinogenicity data indicate the possibility of enhanced skin cancer risk with 5-MOP. Thus, any advocation of the use of 5-MOP-containing sunscreens should be justified by benefits which outweigh long-term risks.

The recent human 5-MOP photochemoprotection data described may well tilt the risk/benefit analysis of 5-MOP sunscreen use in the direction of benefit. An important question in this respect is whether the 5-MOP-DNA lesions, that may occur in obtaining protection, are of greater or lesser consequence (quantitatively and qualitatively) than solar UVR DNA lesions, such as thymine dimers, that may be inhibited by 5-MOP photochemoprotection. Such studies have not been done. Some investigations have been done with 8-MOP in human skin. There is indirect evidence that 8-MOP/DNA lesions may persist for up to 72 hours (69), although the experimental design used did not permit the identification of the location of these lesions; viz the epidermis or the dermis. More recently, monoclonal antibodies for 8-MOP/DNA lesions have shown the presence of 8-MOP nuclear lesions in keratinocytes in vitro and in vivo (70,71).

For the moment, the data suggest that there is a fine balance between inhibiting the photocarcinogenic potential of 5-MOP by sunscreens but, at the same time, maintaining its photochemoprotective potential. There would be no point in adding 5-MOP to a preparation if its protective efficacy was totally inhibited by the concentration of sunscreen present. It is not known if the sunscreen merely reduces the effective concentration of 5-MOP (e.g., is 25 ppm 5-MOP equivalent to 10 ppm in the presence of a sunscreen?) or if the inhibitory effects are dependent on photobiological endpoint. Such would be expected if mechanisms, action spectra, threshold doses, time courses, interactions with other wavelengths and the effects of exposure regime vary with endpoint.

VI. CONCLUSIONS

The concern about the use of 5-MOP in sunscreens is justified. However, risk has been assessed on animal models incapable of showing potential benefit of pigmentation. It is clear that UVB sunscreens act as highly effective anticarcinogens with respect to 5-MOP photocarcinogenicity. The results from the human photochemoprotection studies are encouraging and suggest that the judicious use of 5-MOP-containing sunscreens may have an important role in reducing solar radiation-induced DNA damage in skin. Such damage is widely believed to be the first step in skin cancer development. Given that the potential benefits of photochemoprotection are major, it is important that further research is carried out on the relationship of risk to benefit of 5-MOP-containing sunscreens.

ACKNOWLEDGMENTS

The authors work on 5-MOP was funded by Laboratoires Goupil (now Laboratoires Bergaderm).

REFERENCES

1. Roelandts, R., Vanhee, J., Bonamie, A., Kerkhofs, L., and Degreef, H. A survey of ultraviolet absorbers in commercially available sun products. *Inter. J. Dermatol., 22*:247–255 (1983).
2. Pathak, M. A. Sunscreens: Topical and systemic approaches for protection of human skin against harmful effects of solar radiation. *J. Am. Acad. Dermatol., 7*:285–312 (1982).

3. Hölzle, E., Plewig, G., Hofmann, C., and Roser-Maass, E. Polymorphous light eruption. *J. Am. Acad. Dermatol., 7*:111–125 (1982).
4. McFadden, N. UVA sensitivity and topical photoprotection in polymorphous light eruption. *Photodermatology, 1*:76–78 (1984).
5. Kligman, L. H., Akin, F. J., and Kligman, A. M. Sunscreens prevent ultraviolet photocarcinogenesis. *J. Am. Acad. Dermatol., 3*:30–35 (1980).
6. Kligman, L. H. and Kligman, A. M. The nature of photoageing: Its prevention and repair. *Photodermatology, 3*:215–227 (1986).
7. Plastow, S. R., Harrison, J. A., and Young, A. R. Early changes in dermal collagen of mice exposed to chronic UVB and the effects of a UVB sunscreen. *J. Invest. Dermatol., 91*:590–592 (1988).
8. Slaper, H. and Van der Leun, J. C. The use of sunscreens against long-term sun-damage, *Hazards of Light—Myths and Realities: Eye and Skin* (J. Cronley-Dillon, E. S. Rosen, J. Marshall, eds.), Pergamon Press, New York (1986), pp. 125–132.
9. MacKie, R. A., Elwood, J. M., and Hawk, J. L. M. Links between exposure to ultraviolet radiation and skin cancer. *J. Royal Coll. Phys., 21*:91–96 (1987).
10. van Weelden, H., and van der Leun, J. C. UV-A induced tumors in pigmented and albino hairless mice, *Human Exposure to Ultraviolet Radiation: Risks and Regulations* (W. F. Passchier and B. F. M. Bosnjakovic, eds.), Elsevier Science Publishers B.V., Amsterdam (1987), pp. 45–52.
11. Ohme, C. Über die Zusamensetzung des Bergamottols. *Ann. Chem., 31*: 316–321 (1839).
12. Cieri, U. R. Characterization of the steam nonvolatile residue of bergamot oil and some other essential oils. *J. Am. Off. Anal. Chem., 52*:719–728 (1969).
13. Forlot, P. Possible cancer hazard associated with 5-methoxypsoralen in suntan preparation. *Br. Med. J., 280*:648 (1980).
14. Freund, E. Über bischer noch nicht beschriebene kunstliche Hautverfarbungen. *Derm. Wschr., 63*:931–936 (1916).
15. Parrish, J. A., Fitzpatrick, T. B., Tanenbaum, L., and Pathak, M. A. Photochemotherapy of psoriasis with oral methoxsalen and longwave ultraviolet light. *N. Engl. J. Med., 291*:1207–1211 (1974).
16. Dall'Acqua, F., Terbojevich, M., Marciani, S., Vedaldi, D., and Recher, M. Investigations of the dark interaction between furocoumarins and DNA. *Chem. Biol. Interactions, 21*:103–115 (1978).
17. Sa E Melo, T., Morliere, P., Santus, R., and Dubertret, L. Photoreactivity of 5-methoxypsoralen with calf thymus DNA upon excitation in the UVA. *Photobiochem. Photobiophys., 7*:121–131 (1984).
18. Dall'Acqua, F., Marciani, S., and Rodighiero, G. The action spectrum of xanthotoxin and bergapten for the photoreaction with native DNA. *Z. Naturforsch., 24b*:667–671 (1969).
19. Dall'Acqua, F., Marciani, S., Vedaldi, D., and Rodighiero, G. Skin photosensitization and cross-linkings formation in native DNA by furocoumarins. *Z. Naturforsch., 29c*:635–636 (1974).

20. Averbeck, D. Photochemistry and photobiology of psoralens. *Proc. Jpn. Soc. Invest. Dermatol., 8*:52–73 (1984).

21. Ashwood-Smith, M. J., Poulton, G. A., Barker, M., and Mildenberger, M. 5-Methoxypsoralen, an ingredient in several suntan preparations, has lethal mutagenic and clastogenic properties. *Nature, 285*:407–409 (1980).

22. Urbach, F. Modification of ultraviolet carcinogenesis by photoactive agents. *J. Invest. Dermatol., 32*:373–378 (1959).

23. Forbes, P. D., Davies, R. E., and Urbach, F. Phototoxicity and photocarcinogenesis: Comparative effects of anthracene and 8-methoxysoralen in the skin of mice. *Food Cosmet. Toxicol., 14*:303–306 (1976).

24. Stern, R. S., Laird, N., Melski, J., Parrish, J. A., Fitzpatrick, T. B., and Bleich, H. L. Cutaneous squamous-cell carcinoma in patients treated with PUVA. *N. Engl. J. Med., 310*:1156–1161 (1984).

25. Henseler, T., Christophers, E., Hönigsmann, H., Wolff, K., and nineteen other investigators. Skin tumors in the European PUVA study. *J. Am. Acad. Dermatol., 16*:106–116 (1987).

26. Gibbs, N. K., Hönigsmann, H., and Young, A.R. PUVA treatment strategies and cancer risk. *Lancet*, Jan. 18:150–151 (1986).

27. Hönigsmann, H., Jaschke, E., Gschnait, F., Brenner, W., Fritsch, P., and Wolff, K. 5-Methoxypsoralen (Bergapten) in photochemotherapy of psoriasis. *Br. J. Dermatol., 101*:369–378 (1979).

28. Mezzadra, G., Guarneri, B., Grupper, C., and Forlot, P. Effects of chronic field exposure of humans to bergapten, *Psoralens in Cosmetics and Dermatology* (J. Cahn, P. Forlot, C. Grupper, A. Meybeck, and F. Urbach, eds.), Pergamon Press, Paris (1981), pp. 383–386.

29. 5-Methoxypsoralen. *IARC Monographs on the evaluation of the carcinogenic risk of chemicals to humans 40*:327–347 (1986).

30. Zajdela, F. and Bisagni, E. 5-Methoxypsoralen, the melanogenic additive in sun-tan preparations, is tumorigenic in mice exposed to 365 nm u.v. radiation. *Carcinogenesis, 2*:121–127 (1981).

31. Young, A. R., Magnus, I. A., Davies, A. C., and Smith, N. P. A comparison of the phototumorigenic potential of 8-MOP and 5-MOP in hairless albino mice exposed to solar simulated radiation. *Br. J. Dermatol., 108*:507–518 (1983).

32. Abel, G. Chromosome damage induced in human lymphocytes by 5-methoxypsoralen and 8-methoxypsoralen plus UV-A. *Mutat. Res., 190*:63–68 (1987).

33. Connor, M. J. and Lowe, N. J. The induction of erythema, edema, and the polyamine synthesis enzymes ornithine decarboxylase and S-adenosyl-L-methionine decarboxylase in hairless mouse skin by psoralens and longwave ultraviolet light. *Photochem. Photobiol., 39*:787–792 (1984).

34. O'Brien, T. G. The induction of ornithine decarboxylase as an early, possibly obligatory, event in mouse skin carcinogenesis. *Cancer Res., 36*:2644–2653 (1976).

35. Slaga, T. G. Mechanisms involved in two-stage carcinogenesis in mouse skin, *Mechanisms of Tumor Promotion Volume II: Tumor Promotion and Skin*

Carcinogenesis (T. J. Slaga, ed.), CRC Press Inc., Boca Raton, FL (1984), pp. 1–16.

36. Cartwright, L. E. and Walter, J. F. Psoralen-containing sunscreen is tumorigenic in hairless mice. *J. Am. Acad. Dermatol., 8*:830–836 (1983).

37. Walter, J. F., Gange, R. W., and Mendelson, I. R. Psoralen-containing sunscreen induces phototoxicity and epidermal ornithine decarboxylase activity. *J. Am. Acad. Dermatol., 6*:1022–1027 (1982).

38. Gibbs, N. K., Young, A. R., and Magnus, I. A. Failure of UVR dose reciprocity for skin tumorigenesis in hairless mice treated with 8-methoxypsoralen. *Photochem. Photobiol., 42*:39–42 (1985).

39. Young, A. R., Gibbs, N. K., and Magnus, I. A. Modification of 5-methoxypsoralen phototumorigenesis by UVB sunscreens: A statistical and histologic study in the hairless albino mouse. *J. Invest. Dermatol., 89*:611–617 (1987).

40. Young, A. R. and Walker, S. L. Experimental photocarcinogenesis of psoralens, *Psoralens: Past, Present and Future of Photochemoprotection and Other Biological Activities*, (T. B. Fitzpatrick, P. Forlot, M. A. Pathak, and F. Urbach, eds.), John Libbey Eurotext, Montrouge, France (1989), pp. 357–366.

41. Walker, S. L. and Young, A. R. A possible animal model for the role of induced pigmentation in photocarcinogenesis. *Br. J. Dermatol., 113*:787 (1985).

42. Saettone, M. F., Trambusti, M., and Giannaccini, B. Inhibition de l'action phototoxique du bergaptène par des filtre UV-A. *Int. J. Cosmet. Sci., 5*: 201–213 (1983).

43. Cripps, D. J., Lowe, N. J., and Lerner, A. B. Action spectra of topical psoralens: A re-evaluation. *Br. J. Dermatol., 107*:77–82 (1982).

44. Young, A. R. and Magnus, I. A. An action spectrum for 8-MOP induced sunburn cells in mammalian epidermis. *Br. J. Dermatol., 104*:541–548 (1981).

45. Kaidbey, K. H. An action spectrum for 8-methoxypsoralen-sensitized inhibition of DNA synthesis in vivo. *J. Invest. Dermatol., 85*:98–101 (1985).

46. Gasparro, F. P., Berger, C. L., and Edelson, R. L. Effect of monochromatic UVA light and 8-methoxypsoralen on human lymphocyte response to mitogen. *Photodermatology, 1*:10–17 (1984).

47. Baydoun, S. A. and Young, A. R. An action spectrum for lethal photosensitization of *Candida albicans* by 8-MOP after low-dose broad-band UV-A irradiation; an action spectrum for 8-MOP 4′,5′-monoadducts? *Photochem. Photobiol., 46*:311–314 (1987).

48. Young, A. R., Walker, S. L., and Garmyn, M. G. A first approach to an action spectrum for 8-MOP phototumorigenesis in mice. *J. Invest. Dermatol., 90*:175–178 (1988).

49. Young, A. R. and Barth, J. Comparative studies on the photosensitizing potency of 5-methoxypsoralen and 8-methoxypsoralen as measured by cytolysis in *Paramecium caudatum* and *Tetrahymena pyriformis*, and growth inhibition and survival in *Candida albicans*. *Photochem. Photobiol., 35*: 83–88 (1982).

50. Nakayama, Y., Morikawa, F., Fukuda, M., Hamano, M., Toda, K., and Pathak, M. A. Monochromatic radiation and its application—laboratory studies on the mechanism of erythema and pigmentation induced by psoralen, *Sunlight and Man* (T. B. Fitzpatrick, M. A. Pathak, L. C. Harber, M. Seiji, and A. Kukita, eds.), University of Tokyo Press, Tokyo (1974), pp. 591–611.

51. Morliére, P., Avice, O., Sa E Melo, T., Dubertret, L., Giraud, M., and Santus, R. A study of the photochemical properties of some cinnamate sunscreens by steady state and laser flash photolysis. *Photochem. Photobiol., 36*:395–399 (1982).

52. Bensasson, R. V., Land, E. J., and Salet, C. Triplet excited state of furocoumarins: Reaction with nucleic acid bases and amino acids. *Photochem. Photobiol., 27*:273–280 (1978).

53. Zaynoun, S., Konrad, K., Gschnait, F., and Wolff, K. The pigmentary response to photochemotherapy. *Acta Dermatven, 57*:431–440 (1977).

54. Kenny, J. A. Vitiligo treated by psoralens. *Arch. Dermatol., 103*:475–480 (1971).

55. Brenner, W. and Gschnait, F. The value of topical sunscreens containing psoralens. *Arch. Dermatol. Res., 267*:189–190 (1980).

56. Tronnier, H. and Agache, P. Field trial on suntan products containing bergamot oil in Tunisia, *Psoralens in Cosmetics and Dermatology* (J. Cahn, P. Forlot, C. Grupper, A. Meybeck, and F. Urbach, eds.), Pergamon Press, Paris (1981), pp. 411–417.

57. Sigafoes, R. Evaluation of the tanning potential of topical sunscreens containing psoralens, *Psoralens in Cosmetics and Dermatology* (J. Cahn, P. Forlot, C. Grupper, A. Meybeck, and F. Urbach, eds.), Pergamon Press, Paris (1981), pp. 419–426.

58. Imbrie, J. D., Daniels, F. Bergeron, L., Hopkins, C. E., and Fitzpatrick, T. B. Increased erythema threshold six weeks after a single exposure to sunlight plus oral methoxsalen. *J. Invest. Derm., 32*:331–337 (1959).

59. Cripps, D. J. Natural and artificial photoprotection. *J. Invest. Dermatol., 76*:154–157 (1981).

60. Gschnait, F., Brenner, W., and Wolff, K. Photoprotective effect of a psoralen-UVA-induced tan. *Arch. Dermatol. Res., 263*:181–188 (1978).

61. Gschnait, F., Hönigsmann, H., Brenner, W., Fritsch, P., and Wolff, K. Induction of UV light tolerance by PUVA in patients with polymorphous light eruption. *Br. J. Dermatol., 99*:293–295 (1978).

62. Sambuco, C. P., Forbes, P. D., Davies, R. E., and Urbach, F. Protective value of skin tanning induced by ultraviolet radiation plus a sunscreen containing bergamot oil. *J. Soc. Cosmet. Chem., 38*:11–19 (1987).

63. Young, A. R. The sunburn cell. *Photodermatology, 4*:127–134 (1987).

64. Young, A. R., Potten, C. S., Chadwick, C. A., Murphy, G. M., and Cohen, A. J. Inhibition of UV radiation-induced DNA damage by a 5-methoxypsoralen tan in human skin. *Pigment Cell Res., 1*:350–354 (1988).

65. Potten, C. S., Chadwick, C. A., Young, A. R., Murphy, G. M., and Cohen,

A. J. A 5-methoxypsoralen-induced tan protects against DNA damage from a subsequent exposure to solar simulated radiation in human skin, *Psoralens: Past, Present and Future of Photochemoprotection and other Biological Activities* (T. B. Fitzpatrick, P. Forlot, M. A. Pathak, and F. Urbach, eds.), John Libby Eurotext, Montrouge, France (1989).

66. Ashwood-Smith, M. J. Possible cancer hazard associated with 5-methoxysoralen in suntan preparations. *Br. Med. J.*, *2*:1144 (1979).

67. Hook, I. Possible cancer hazard associated with 5-methoxypsoralen in suntan preparations. *Br. Med. J.*, *280*:1537–1538 (1980).

68. Natarajan, A. T., Verdegaal-Immerzeel, E. A. M., Ashwood-Smith, M. J., and Poulton, G. A. Chromosomal damage induced by furocoumarins and UVA in hamster and human cells including cells from patients with ataxia telangiectasia and xeroderma pigmentosum. *Mutat. Res.*, *84*:113–124 (1981).

69. Gange, R. W., Levins, P., Murray, J., Anderson, R., and Parrish, J. A. Prolonged skin photosensitization induced by methoxalen and subphototoxic UVA irradiation. *J. Invest. Dermatol.*, *82*:219–222 (1984).

70. Yang, X. Y., DeLeo, V., and Santella, R. M. Immunological detection and visualization of 8-methoxypsoralen-DNA photoadducts. *Cancer Res.*, *47*: 2451–2455 (1987).

71. Yang, X. Y., Gasparro, F. P., DeLeo, V. A., and Santella, R. M. 8-Methoxypsoralen-DNA adducts in patients treated with 8-methoxypsoralen and ultraviolet A light. *J. Invest. Dermatol.*, *92*:59–63 (1989).

8

Contact Sensitization and Photocontact Sensitization of Sunscreening Agents

SYDNEY H. DROMGOOLE *Herbert Laboratories, Santa Ana, California*

HOWARD I. MAIBACH *University of California Medical Center, San Francisco, California*

I. INTRODUCTION

Sunscreens can be classified into two major types: chemical and physical sunscreens (1). Physical sunscreens such as titanium dioxide and zinc oxide reduce the amount of light penetrating the skin by creating a physical barrier that reflects, scatters, or physically blocks the ultraviolet light reaching the skin surface. Chemical sunscreens, on the other hand, reduce the amount of light reaching the stratum corneum by absorbing the radiation. Examples of chemical sunscreens include para amino benzoic acid (PABA) and PABA derivatives such as Padimate O, cinnamates, benzophenones, salicylate derivatives, and dibenzoylmethane derivatives.

Because chemical sunscreens are applied topically to the skin in relatively high concentrations (up to 26%), contact sensitization can occur. Similarly, because these chemicals absorb radiation, they have the potential to cause photosensitization. Both types of sensitization can occur with not only the various sunscreening agents but also with excipients such as emulsifiers, antioxidants, and preservatives that are included in the various hydroalcoholic lotions, ointments, oil-in-water or water-in-oil emulsions.

Despite extensive sunscreen use for several decades, there have been relatively few published reports of sunscreen-induced side effects, including allergic/photoallergic reactions, but we probably have inadequate data to accurately predict the degree of hypersensitivity to sunscreening agents due to the lack of a well-developed adverse reaction reporting system.

Reprinted with permission from the *Journal of the American Academy of Dermatology*, Mosby Year Book, 1990.

This chapter reviews the reports of contact sensitization and photocontact sensitization induced by various sunscreening agents currently in use in the United States and discusses the strategies for patch and photopatch testing, as well as immediate-type testing.

II. LITERATURE REPORTS

Published reports of contact and photocontact sensitization and contact urticaria induced by sunscreening agents are listed in Table 1. Representatives of all major sunscreen categories including PABA derivatives, anthranilates, salicylates, cinnamates, and benzophenones have caused allergic reactions (2-52).

A. Para Amino Benzoic Acid (PABA)

In 1976, Willis (53) suggested that the sensitization potential of *p*-amino benzoic acid was minimal. Wennersten et al. (7) reported that a total of 73/1883 (3.9%) subjects tested with 5% PABA in alcohol in the Scandinavian Standard Photopatch Tray had either allergic or photoallergic responses to PABA. These subjects represent 73% of the total number of subjects with contact and photocontact sensitization to PABA (Table 1). The use of PABA as a sunscreening agent in Europe and the United States has decreased significantly in recent years. PABA has been replaced by ester derivatives such as Padimate O that, unlike PABA, are not water soluble and tend to remain on the surface layer with less than 10% penetrating the corneum even after 24 hours (47). These PABA esters appear to be less sensitizing than PABA; however, there is no "hard" data to substantiate this impression.

B. PABA Derivatives

Sensitization to glyceryl PABA was first reported by Sulzberger et al. (54), and during the next 30 years additional reports appeared (3, 15-19, 21, 50). Many of the cases of glyceryl PABA sensitization showed uniform strong reactions to benzocaine, suggesting that the sensitization may be due to the presence of impurities in the glyceryl PABA. This suggestion was first made by Fisher (19) and has since been confirmed (20, 22, 42, 55, 56). Benzocaine impurities (1-18%) occurred in many commercial sources of glyceryl PABA. Thus many of the early reports of contact allergy to glyceryl PABA may have falsely implicated glyceryl PABA as the sensitizer. Thune (8) recently reported two cases of allergic/photoallergic reactions to glyceryl PABA in which there was no reaction to benzocaine, suggesting true allergy to the PABA derivative. However, no allergic responses were observed when these subjects were patched with glyceryl PABA which had been purified via high-pressure liquid chromatography (56). This suggests the presence of an, as yet, unknown impurity (or impurities) other than

Table 1 Contact and Photocontact Sensitization to Sunscreening Agents

Chemical	Number of subjects with contact dermatitis	Number of subjects with photocontact dermatitis	Total
p-Amino benzoic acid (PABA)	49	52	101
Glyceryl amino benzoate (Glyceryl PABA)	28	6	34
Amyl-*p*-dimethylamino benzoate (Padimate A)	6	14	20
Octyl-dimethyl PABA (Padimate O)	11	2	13
Ethoxyethyl methoxy-cinnamate (Cinoxate)	5	10	15
Digalloyl trioleate	1	0	1
Oxybenzone	2	12	14
Dioxybenzone	2	0	2
Sulisobenzone	3	2	5
Homosalate	2	2	4
2-Phenylbenzimidazole-5-sulfonic acid	4	2	6
Butyl-methoxydibenzoyl-methane (avobenzone)[a]	6	8	14
Isopropyl-methoxy-dibenzoylmethane (Eusolex 8020)[b]	34	15	49
Hydroxymethoxy methyl benzophenone (Mexenone)[b]	9	1	10
3-(4-Methyl-benzylidene camphor (Eusolex 6300)[b]	16	5	21

[a]Avobenzone is the United States Adopted Name (USAN) of this chemical. It is also known as Parsol 1789, the Cosmetics, Toiletry and Fragrances Association (CTFA) name.
[b]Not an FDA-approved sunscreening agent.
Source: Refs. 2–52.

benzocaine as the sensitization source. The glyceryl PABA scenario underscores the importance of utilizing purified raw materials in the manufacture of consumer products such as sunscreening agents and the need for careful interpretation of patch test results.

Other PABA derivatives that have caused sensitization/photocontact sensitization include octyl dimethyl PABA (Padimate O), amyl dimethyl PABA (Padimate A), and ethyl dihydroxy PABA. The number of case reports of sensitization/photocontact sensitization with Padimate O is less than that reported with PABA and glyceryl PABA suggesting a lower sensitization potential with this derivative. This may be because Padimate O is not a true PABA ester since it does not contain the NH_2 grouping present in glyceryl PABA, PABA, and benzocaine (20).

Padimate A also lacks the NH_2 grouping and, although it was included in the proposed sunscreen monograph (1) as a safe and effective sunscreening agent, this derivative can cause phototoxicity (45,57) and may have accounted for the erythemal response observed by Katz (46) 30 minutes after sun exposure. This compound is no longer used in sunscreens in the United States. In addition to finding benzocaine impurities in the glyceryl PABA raw materials Bruze et al. (55) also found that some PABA esters contain 0.2 to 4.5% PABA. It is therefore possible that these PABA impurities may account for some of the reports of sensitization to the PABA derivatives.

C. Salicylates

There are only two cases of contact allergy and two reports of photocontact allergy to homomenthyl salicylate in the literature (10,25) and no reports of sensitization to octyl salicylate, the major salicylate derivative incorporated in many sunscreens.

D. Cinnamates

Cinnamates are chemically related to or are found in balsam of Peru, balsam of Tolu, coca leaves, cinnamic acid, cinnamic aldehyde and cinnamon oil, ingredients used in perfumes, topical medications, cosmetics, and flavoring. Thune reported eight cases of sensitivity to cinnamates, two cases of photoallergy to 2-ethoxyethyl-*p*-cinnamate, and six subjects with contact allergy to other cinnamates such as amyl cinnamaldehyde, amyl cinnamic acid, and cinnamon oil (8). Cross-sensitization among cinnamon derivatives has been reported (58).

E. Benzophenones

There have been twelve reported cases of photocontact allergy (8, 10, 13, 38, 43, 44) and two cases of contact allergy (9, 26) to oxybenzone, and three reports of contact allergy (5, 29) and two reports of photocontact allergy to sulisobenzone (10). Benzophenone-10 (Mexenone), a benzophenone derivative not used in sunscreens in the United States, can also cause contact and photo-contact dermatitis (8, 30, 36, 49).

F. Dibenzoylmethanes

Dibenzoylmethane derivatives such as isopropyldibenzoylmethane (Eusolex 8020) and butyl dibenzoylmethane (avobenzone) have been incorporated in European sunscreens as UVA absorbers since 1980 (57). Instances of contact allergy/photoallergy to the dibenzoylmethanes or sunscreens and lipsticks containing these derivatives have been reported, although the majority of these reports have been associated with the isopropyl derivative (11, 27, 28, 31–33, 51, 52). As a consequence of these adverse reactions to Eusolex 8020, several manufacturers of products that contained this ingredient have stopped incorporating this derivative into their products (51, 52). On the other hand, there have been fewer reports of contact allergy/photoallergy to the butyl dibenzoylmethane derivative, avobenzone (11,27,28,30,31). It is possible that some of these reactions to avobenzone may have been cross-reactions resulting from prior exposure to the isopropyl derivative (27, 28, 30). Greater utilization of these compounds with appropriate testing should help clarify their relative sensitization potential.

G. Camphor Derivatives

3-(4-Methyl-benzylidene) camphor (Eusolex 6300) is a sunscreening agent used extensively in Europe, often in combination with Eusolex 8020, but it is not approved for use in the United States. There have been several reports of allergic and photoallergic reactions to sunscreens containing this agent (27, 30, 32, 35, 37, 52).

H. Miscellaneous

Other chemical sunscreens that have caused allergic reactions include diagalloyl trioleate (12), the glycerol ester of o-aminometa (2,3 dihydroxyproxy) benzoic acid (60), a dioxane derivative (6), and 2-phenyl-5-methyl-benzoazol (witisol) (61). None of these ingredients are approved for use in sunscreens in the United States.

I. Titanium Dioxide

Physical blockers such as titanium dioxide and zinc oxide have the advantage of not being sensitizers, but such agents may be so occlusive that they can cause miliaria (62). It is interesting to note that Kaminester reported that the inclusion of titanium dioxide in a PABA sunscreen blocked the appearance of photoallergy (63). It is possible that the reflection and scattering of light by titanium dioxide reduced the amount of UV light that penetrated the skin and elicited the photoallergic response.

J. Excipients

Although the objective of this chapter is to discuss sensitization to sunscreening agents, it is important to point out that contact allergy can also be caused by excipients included in the formulations. These chemicals include mineral oil, petrolatum, isopropyl esters, lanolin derivatives, aliphatic alcohols, triglycerides, fatty acids, waxes, propylene glycol, emulsifiers, thickeners, preservatives, and fragrances. Table 2 lists some of the excipients used in sunscreen formulations

Table 2 Excipients That Can Cause Contact or Photocontact Dermatitis

Avocado oil
t-Butyl alcohol
Methyl paraben
Phenyl dimethicone
Solvent red 1
Solvent red 3
Triethanolamine stearate
Benzyl alcohol
Cetylstearyl alcohol
Sorbitan sesquiolate
Imidazolidinyl urea (Germall 115)
Methylisothiazolinone/methylchloroisothiazolinone (Kathon CG)
Glyceryl monostearate
6-Acetoxy-2,4-dimethyl-m-dioxane
Carbowaxes
Ethyl alcohol
Glycerol
Isopropyl alcohol
Isopropyl myristate
Petrolatum
Stearyl alcohol

Sources: From Refs. 62–76.

that have caused allergic reactions (64–76). A more extensive list of vehicle constituents in cosmetics that can cause allergic responses has been published (64). A recent study by de Groot et al. (74) indicated that preservatives, fragrances, and emulsifiers are the main classes of ingredients responsible for cosmetic allergy, with Kathon CG (a mixture of methylisothiazolinone/methylchloroisothiazolinone) producing contact allergic reactions in 27.7% of subjects tested. In view of the potential to cause sensitization, the Cosmetic Ingredient Review (CIR) Expert Panel in the United States has recently requested additional patch testing of Kathon CG (72).

Many sunscreens available in the United States provide a complete list of ingredients including the excipients. The listing of all ingredients in sunscreens should be encouraged so that consumers, especially those with known sensitivities to chemicals, are fully informed about the composition of the formulation prior to the purchase and application of the product to the skin.

III. CROSS-SENSITIZATION REACTIONS

Cross-sensitization reactions are defined as additional allergic responses that occur in one or more compounds (78, 79). The allergen causing the primary reaction is the primary sensitizer, while secondary allergens are those compounds that can cause cross-sensitization. In general, these compounds have similar chemical structures or are metabolized to chemical structures similar to the primary allergen. However, in many instances it is difficult to determine which allergen is the primary allergen.

Cross-sensitization reactions with other sunscreens as well as with chemicals with similar chemical structures have been reported but are uncommon. Table 3 summarizes the published reports of cross-sensitization among the sunscreening agents. Many sunscreens containing PABA or PABA derivatives in the United States include a statement in the labeling that the use of the product is contraindicated in subjects who have known sensitivities to *p*-phenyldiamine, aniline, procaine, benzocaine, sulfonamides, and several azo dyes. These contraindications were based on the early studies by Meltzer and Baer (16), and Curtis and Crawford (17) with glyceryl PABA. It is now established by Fisher (19, 20, 35) and more recently by Bruze et al. (55, 56) that benzocaine and possibly other impurities may have been responsible for some of the reports of cross-sensitization associated with glyceryl PABA. It is therefore possible that some of the other reported cross-sensitizations to glyceryl PABA may also have been due to cross-reactions to benzocaine and not to glyceryl PABA. This possibility underscores the need to insure that the reported sensitization of various chemicals is due to the chemical and not to impurities. This has been discussed by Bruze et al. (56) and is important for several reasons: (1) the subjects may be advised to

Table 3 Cross-Sensitization to Other Chemicals and Sunscreens

Sunscreen	Cross-sensitizer(s)	Reference
p-Amino benzoic acid (PABA)	Padimate O, oxybenzone	(4) (9)
	Glyceryl PABA	(3) (23)
	Sulfonamides	(54)
	p-Phenylenediamine (PPD)	(8) (78)
	Benzocaine	(3) (33)
	Padimate A	(3) (8)
	Padimate O	(3) (8) (9)
	Glyceryl PABA	(3)
Cinoxate	Cinnamaldehyde	(6)
	p-Methoxyisoamylcinnamate	(6)
	Balsam of Peru	(4)
	Benzyl cinnamate	(4)
	Methyl cinnamate	(4)
	Cinnamyl alcohol	(4)
Oxybenzone	Dioxybenzone	(13) (14)
	p-Phenylenediamine	(44)

Padimate O	p-Amino benzoic acid	(3) (8) (9)
	Cinoxate	(33)
	Isobutyl PABA	(47)
Padimate A	p-Amino benzoic acid	(8)
Isopropyl-methoxydibenzoylmethane (Eusolex 8020)	t-Butyl methoxydibenzoylmethane (avobenzone)	(27) (28) (30) (31)
Glyceryl PABA	Sulfonamides	(15) (16) (50)
	Benzocaine	(16) (17) (19) (20) (21) (42)
	Procaine	(15) (19) (20)
	Aniline	(15) (17) (19)
	p-Diphenyldiamine	(15) (17) (19) (20)
	PABA	(8) (15) (17) (19) (20)
	Picric acid	(16)
	Azodye A	(16)
	Butyl aminobenzoate (butesin)	(16) (17)
	Saccharin	(16)
Sulisobenzone	Oxybenzone	(29)

avoid the wrong substances and (2) effective and safe compounds may be prematurely withdrawn from the market place.

It is also interesting to note that the number of cross-sensitizations to octyl dimethyl PABA (Padimate O), the most common and widely used UVB absorber in sunscreens, is rare. Camarasa and Serra-Baldrich (9) reported one subject sensitive to PABA who also reacted to Padimate O and oxybenzone while one subject sensitive to Padimate O also reacted to PABA. Rietschel and Lewis (25) reported that two subjects who had contact dermatitis to homosalate were not sensitive to PABA, menthyl anthranilate, cinnamates, or PABA esters. Fisher noted that four patients with sensitivity to benzocaine and glyceryl PABA did not show cross-reactions to Padimate O or Padimate A (20), while Thune (8) reported that cross-sensitization did not occur between Padimate O and Padimate A, but all subjects sensitive to the PABA derivatives were also sensitive to p-amino benzoic acid.

It is of great clinical relevance to the sensitized patient to know if PABA and its esters cross-react in either allergic or photoallergic dermatitis. Adequate quantitative data is needed; for the moment, it appears that true cross-reactions (not due to contaminants) do not routinely occur. Patch and photopatch testing with each of the sunscreens could be used to define this problem as efficiently as possible. Even when such testing is negative, we suggest cautious application to an exposed noncosmetic area for 5 days prior to widespread application.

Cross-sensitization to the cinnamate derivative Cinoxate included cinnamic aldehyde, p-methoxyisoamylcinnamate, balsam of Peru, benzyl cinnamate, cinnamyl alcohol, and methyl cinnamate (4,6).

Recently de Groot et al. (30,31) reported on the cross-sensitization among the dibenzoylmethane derivatives used in European sunscreens. Several subjects sensitive to Eusolex 8020 were also sensitive to avobenzone. Schauder and Ippen (28) have reported that in Europe (photo)allergic reactions to Eusolex 8020 are more frequent than to the t-butyl derivative, avobenzone. These authors also noted that there have been no instances of subjects who reacted to avobenzone but not to Eusolex 8020, whereas the reverse situation is not infrequently observed.

It has been noted recently that contact dermatitis and photoallergic contact dermatitis to different sunscreens can occur simultaneously (28). This phenomenon can be explained by a combination of cross-reaction and coupling allergy.

IV. SUNSCREEN SENSITIZATION IN PHOTODERMATOSES

MacLeod and Frain-Bell have emphasized the importance of using a sunscreen that is appropriate for the action spectrum of the patient's photodermatoses (80). However, there is increasing evidence that some subjects with photodermatoses such as chronic actinic dermatitis, polymorphous light eruption, or persistent light reactions not only have increased sensitivity to light but also increased sensitivity to chemicals (81–83). Thune and Eeg-Larsen (81) found that of 18 males with persistent light reactivity, 17 showed allergic reactions. Of these, 12 were positive photopatch test reactions and 11 were contact allergic reactions. Four of these subjects had positive patch tests to sunscreens: two to PABA, one to oxybenzone, and one to Padimate A. In addition, ten subjects with polymorphous light eruption exhibited positive photopatch or contact allergic reactions. Two subjects exhibited photosensitivity to PABA and one subject was sensitive to two cinnamate derivatives.

Many of the reports included in Table 1 involved subjects with various photosensitivities. These photosensitivities are listed in Table 4. Photosensitive subjects who require protection from the sun need to be patch and photopatch tested to the various sunscreening agents to determine the specific sensitizers/photosensitizers. Once the offending agents have been identified, the subject can eliminate the sunscreens that contain these chemicals, and their presumably endogenous photosensitivity may be easier to manage (84).

Of course, it is possible that some subjects may not be sensitive to the active sunscreening agents but to one or more of the many excipients included in the sunscreen formulations. In such cases, the selection of a suitable sunscreen is made more difficult, and customized sunscreens eliminating the sensitizing compounds may be necessary to allow subjects to cope with daily living.

Table 4 Photodermatoses That May Be Aggravated by Sunscreening Agents

Atopic dermatitis

Lichen rubeo planus

Polymorphous light eruption (PMLE)

Chronic actinic dermatitis (chronic photosensitive eczema, actinic reticuloid)

Xeroderma pigmentosa (XP)

Persistent light reaction (PLR)

Herpes labialis

Musk ambrette photosensitivity

Idiopathic photosensitivities

Lupus erythematosus (LE)

Phytophotodermatitis

Seborrheic dermatitis

Sources: From Refs. 2, 4, 5, 7, 8, 14, 16, 17, 27, 28, 30, 31, 33, 36, 41, 48, 52, 81.

V. SUNSCREENS IN THE UNITED STATES

There are more than 100 sunscreening preparations currently sold in the United
States. Only 14 of the 21 sunscreen agents included in the proposed sunscreen
monograph are commonly used in sunscreens in the United States (Table 5). One
additional sunscreening agent used in sunscreens that is not included in the proposed FDA sunscreen monograph is *t*-butyl dimethoxydibenzoylmethane (avobenzone). The latter chemical has only been recently approved in the United
States but has been used extensively in sunscreens in Europe for several years. It
is also interesting to note that zinc oxide, included as an inactive ingredient in
the sunscreen monograph, is commonly used as a sunscreening agent.

Table 6 lists examples of the sunscreen formulations sold in the United States
together with the active ingredients and their sun protection factors (SPF)—a
measure of sunscreen protection against sunburn. The table has been subdi-
vided into four categories depending on the number of active sunscreening
chemicals in the formulation. Most of the formulations that are combination
sunscreens contain one or more UVB absorbers and a UVA absorber to provide
much needed protection against the damaging effects of UVA. Several sunscreens also include physical blockers such as titanium dioxide.

Table 5   Approved Sunscreening Agents Used in United States

Aminobenzoic acid (PABA)

2-Ethoxyethyl-*p*-methoxycinnamate (Cinoxate)

Dioxybenzone

Ethyl 4-(bis(hydroxypropyl) aminobenzoate

2-Ethylhexyl 2-cyano-3,3-diphenylacrylate (octocrylene)

Ethylhexyl *p*-methoxycinnamate (Parsol MCX)

Octyl salicylate

Glyceryl PABA

Homomenthyl salicylate (homosalate)

Menthyl anthranilate

Oxybenzone

Octyl dimethyl PABA (Padimate O)

2-Phenylbenzimidazole-5-sulfonic acid

Titanium dioxide

t-Butyl dimethoxy dibenzoylmethane (avobenzone)[a]

---

[a]Not included in the proposed sunscreen monograph (1).
Source: From Ref. 1.

Table 6 Selected Sunscreen Formulations Available in the United States

Trade name	SPF	Active ingredients
Four Sunscreening Ingredients:		
Coppertone (Plough)	30	Padimate O, Parsol MCX, octyl salicylate, oxybenzone
Sundown (Johnson & Johnson)	30	Parsol MCX, octyl salicylate, oxybenzone, titanium dioxide
	20	Padimate O, Parsol MCX, octyl salicylate, oxybenzone
Cancer Garde (Eclipse Labs)	30	Padimate O, Parsol MCX, oxybenzone, titanium dioxide
T/I Screen (T/I Pharmaceuticals)	30+	Parsol MCX, octocrylene, octyl salicylate, oxybenzone
Block Out (Carter Products)	30	Parsol MCX, padimate O, octyl salicylate, oxybenzone
Supershade (Plough)	44	Parsol MCX, padimate O, homosalate, oxybenzone
Three Sunscreening Ingredients:		
Solbar (Person and Covey)	50	Parsol MCX, octocrylene, oxybenzone
PreSun for Kids (Westwood)	39	Parsol MCX, octyl salicylate, oxybenzone
PreSun 29	29	Parsol MCX, octyl salicylate, oxybenzone
Bain de Soleil (Bain de Soleil)	30	Padimate O, Parsol MCX, oxybenzone
Ultrashade (Plough)	23	Padimate O, Parsol MCX, oxybenzone
Total Eclipse (Eclipse Labs)	15	Padimate O, octyl salicylate, oxybenzone
Sundown (Johnson & Johnson)	15	Padimate O, Parsol MCX, oxybenzone
Two Sunscreening Ingredients:		
Supershade (Plough)	8, 15	Parsol MCX, oxybenzone
Coppertone (Plough)	4, 6, 8, 15	Padimate O, oxybenzone
Shade (Plough)	4, 6	Padimate O, oxybenzone
PreSun (Westwood)	8, 15	Padimate O, oxybenzone
Water Babies (Plough)	15	Parsol MCX, oxybenzone

Table 6 (Continued)

Trade name	SPF	Active ingredients
Sundown (Johnson & Johnson)	4, 6, 8	Padimate O, oxybenzone
Block Out (Carter Products)	15	Padimate O, oxybenzone
Photoplex (Herbert Labs)	15+	Padimate O, avobenzone
One Sunscreening Ingredient:		
Coppertone (Plough)	2	Octyl salicylate
Bain de Soleil (Bain de Soleil)	2, 4	Padimate O
Eclipse (Eclipse Labs)	5	Padimate O
Eclipse (Eclipse Labs	10	Glyceryl PABA

In general, as the SPF of the sunscreen formulation increases, the number of active ingredients increases to three or four, and in some cases the total amount of active sunscreens increases up to 26%. Not all formulations list the specific concentrations of the active ingredients, and it is possible that some may contain higher concentrations. As with many chemicals, increasing the concentrations of the active ingredients also increases the likelihood of sensitization (14).

The majority of sunscreens contain octyl dimethyl PABA (Padimate O) as the main UVB absorber. The cinnamate derivative, octyl methoxycinnamate (Parsol MCX), is also used as a UVB absorber.

Most sunscreens with more than one ingredient contain oxybenzone as the additional ingredient. The absorption peak of this compound lies in the UVB region and extends partially into the UVA. Other agents that absorb in the UVA region include sulisobenzone, dioxybenzone, menthyl anthranilate, and avobenzone. The latter chemical having an absorption maximum in the middle of the UVA region (358 nm), has only recently been approved in the United States in one sunscreen formulation (Photoplex, Herbert Laboratories, Santa Ana, CA) (Table 6).

VI. PATCH AND PHOTOPATCH TESTING: CONTACT VERSUS PHOTOCONTACT DERMATITIS

The criteria for separating allergic contact and allergic photocontact dermatitis utilizing patch-testing techniques are imprecise. General criteria and their interpretation are listed in Table 7. Often, the results are not all or none, as implied in the table. Frequently, there is a difference in response intensity, with either the contact or photocontact response being greater. All too infrequently serial dilutions are performed with either the putative antigen or the amount of

Table 7 Patch and Photopatch Testing[a]

Contact test site response	Photocontact test site response	Interpretation
Positive	Positive	Allergic contact dermatitis
Negative	Positive	Photoallergic contact dermatitis
Negative	Negative	Not sensitized

[a]See text for details.

ultraviolet light employed. Until a significant number of patients are so studied, it will be unclear how many of them represent contact versus photocontact sensitization.

A. Light Source

Wennersten et al. (38) recommend that patients with suspected photocontact allergy be phototested prior to implementation of patch testing. The aim of this preliminary light testing is to detect any abnormal sensitivity to UVA and UVB wavebands. It is generally agreed that UVA sources are adequate and sufficient to elicit responses, an important convenience as UVA does not produce erythema in normal fair-skinned subjects until a dose of 20–30 J/cm^2 is delivered. Most photoallergies will be defined with a far smaller dose. Although some data on the dose of light required to elicit a response exists, this remains incomplete and must be studied in context with the dose of antigen and the vehicle. Until the light and antigenic intensities are more fully defined, most physicians are utilizing a PUVA unit, a bank of UVA bulbs in a diagnostic unit or a hot quartz (Kromayer) unit, with an appropriate filter to remove any light with wavelengths below 320 nm (UVB).

The effect of UV irradiation on photopatch test substances in vitro has been reported by Bruze et al. (85). All thirteen photoactive compounds formed photoproducts after UVA irradiation; 8 substances were decomposed by both UVA and UVB radiation; 5 by UVA alone. It is also possible that some patients may require UVB to elicit photoallergic dermatitis. However, since UVB testing is not done routinely, it may be some time before this is clarified.

B. Masked Patch Test

Epstein (86) observed that many patients are so sensitive to light that the dose delivered under an ordinary patch will elicit reactions. He provided details of testing the nonexposed site, utilizing a large light-impermeable black patch applied in a dimly lit room. This precaution remains essential for those decisions of separating the two mechanisms.

C. Antigen Source

Commercial sources of appropriately diluted sunscreen antigens are not presently available in the United States. On request, many thoughtful manufacturers provide patch-test kits of individual ingredients for their products. A "standard" series of sunscreen antigens has been proposed by the International Contact Dermatitis Research Group (ICDRG). In Europe, these test kits are commercially available (Fig. 1). These sunscreen antigens are available in 2% concentrations, although the maximum nonirritating doses of putative antigens in a given vehicle have not been defined. Test concentrations and vehicles for the dermatological testing of many other cosmetic ingredients that may be in sunscreen formulations have been published elsewhere (87).

D. Vehicle

The specific vehicle in which the allergens are dissolved or suspended is very important (88). The ICDRG list (Fig. 1) employs petrolatum as diluent. This vehicle appears to be adequate to elicit reactions in many patients. It is clear, however, that the bioavailability of the antigen may be too limited in some cases. Thus Mathias et al. (23) required ethanol to demonstrate PABA sensitivity, and Schauder and Ippen (28) noted more pronounced test reactions to avobenzone in isopropylmyristate than vaseline. This topic remains an area for study, for instance, optimal vehicle and concentration for each ingredient.

E. Enigmas

Some patients develop sunscreen-induced dermatitis reactions that appear allergic or photoallergic in a morphologic and historic sense, yet fail to demonstrate a positive patch or photopatch test, in spite of seemingly appropriate testing. Such false-negative reactions are more difficult to identify than false-positive reactions (89). Table 8 provides the basic strategy employed in attempting to help these patients. Unfortunately, in some patients, even these extensive manoeuvres fail to elicit the culprit.

F. Excited Skin Syndrome

Many of the reported positives to date, and especially the cross-reaction studies, may well represent false-positives due to the excited skin syndrome. This state of skin hyperirritability often induced by a concomitant dermatitis is responsible for many nonreproducible patch tests. Bruynzeel and Maibach (90) detail strattegies for minimizing such false-positives.

Table 8 Strategy for Identifying the Cause When Routine Patch Testing Is Negative

Intervention	Comment
Increase UVA dose	Avoid UVA erythema; utilize UVA control
Increase concentration of sunscreen	Upper limit of nonirritating dose not completely defined
Alter vehicle	Ethanol has been found to be effective
Test other components	Sunscreen manufacturers often helpful in providing test kits
Add suberythemogenic doses of UVB	
Perform provocative use test on final formulation	
Consider "compound" allergy	

G. Burning and Stinging: Contact Urticaria and Subjective (Sensory) Irritation

Many products, when applied to the face, burn, itch, or sting (29, 91-94). The mechanism may be either subjective (sensory) irritation or contact urticaria. The latter describes a wheal and flare response that occurs within 30 to 60 minutes after cutaneous exposure. This response may be allergic or nonallergic and has been reported with benzophenone (29). It is most likely that the diagnosis is generally missed, as only rarely is immediate type (wheal and flare) testing performed. Von Krogh and Maibach (95) review diagnostic criteria and testing methods. Subjective irritation remains a major factor in decreased use of sunscreens, in other words, patients discontinue use because of discomfort. Much remains to be done to resolve this complication (96).

VII. CONCLUSIONS

The potential of sunscreening agents to cause sensitization is theoretically high because of the high concentrations of these active ingredients in the formulations. However, despite the widespread use of sunscreens, the small number of published reports of contact/photocontact sensitization to these agents suggests that such sensitization is a minimal problem in dermatology. Wennersten et al. (38) reported that the frequency of hypersensitivity to sunscreens in their patient population is about 0.1%, while Nater and De Groot (64) report that the

1-(4-isopropylphenyl)-3-phenyl-1,3-propanediol

CAS number: 63250-25-9

Chemical Structure:

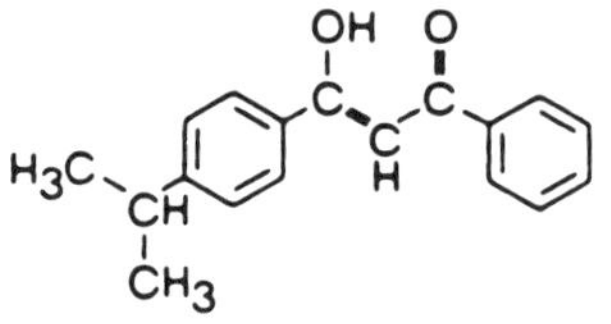

Synonyms: Eusolex 8020, 4-isopropyldibenzoylmethane

UV absorption maximum: 345nm (100)

Usual concentration: 0.5 to 1.5%

(a)

4-t-butyl-4'-methoxy-dibenzoylmethane

CAS number: 70356-09-1

Chemical Structure:

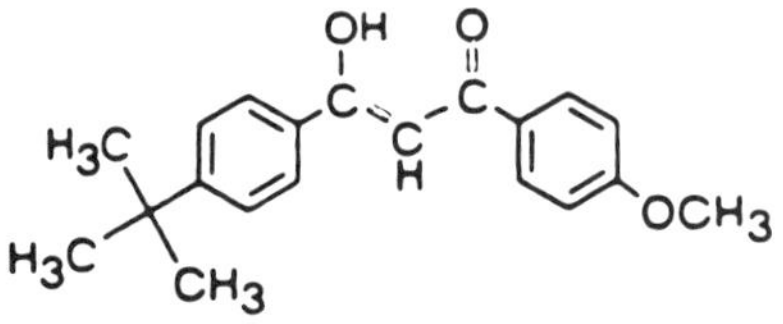

Synonyms: Parsol 1789, Avobenzone, 1-4-(1,1-dimethylethyl)phenyl-3-(4-methoxyphenyl)-1,3-propanedione

UV absorption maximum: 358nm (100)

(b)

Figure 1 Sunscreen antigens available in Europe, 2% concentration in petrolatum. (Note: Sunscreen antigens available from Trolab Company, Hermal Chemie, Hamburg, West Germany.)

p-aminobenzoic acid

CAS number: 150-13-0

Chemical Structure:

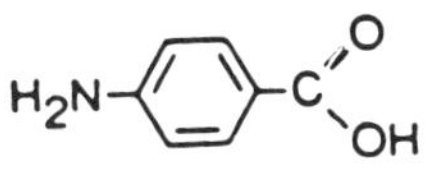

$$H_2N-\left\langle\bigcirc\right\rangle-C\underset{OH}{\overset{O}{<}}$$

Synonyms: PAB, PABA, Papacidium, Vitamin H

UV absorption maximum: 283-289nm (1,100)

Usual concentration: 3% to 5%

(c)

2-Ethylhexyl-p-dimethylaminobenzoate

CAS number: 21245-02-3

Chemical Structure:

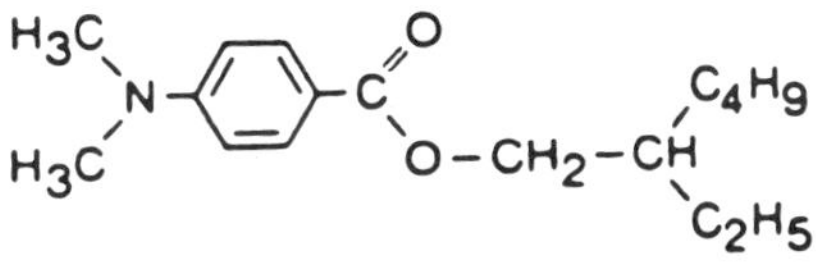

$$\underset{H_3C}{\overset{H_3C}{>}}N-\left\langle\bigcirc\right\rangle-C\underset{O-CH_2-CH\underset{C_2H_5}{\overset{C_4H_9}{<}}}{\overset{O}{<}}$$

Synonyms: Escalol 507, padimate O, Eusolex 6007

UV absorption maximum: 310nm (1,100)

Usual concentration: 0.5 to 5%

(d)

Figure 1 (cont.)

2-Ethylhexyl-p-methoxycinnamate

CAS number: 5466-77-3

Chemical Structure:

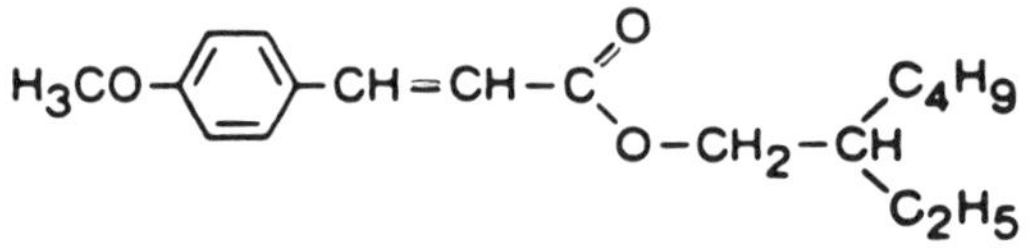

$$H_3CO-\langle\bigcirc\rangle-CH=CH-C{\overset{O}{\underset{O-CH_2-CH}{}}}{\overset{C_4H_9}{\underset{C_2H_5}{}}}$$

Synonyms: Neo-Heliopan AV, Parsol MCX

UV absorption maximum: 310-311nm (1,100)

Usual concentration: Up to 6.5%

(e)

2-Ethoxyethyl-p-methoxycinnamate

CAS number: 104-28-9

Chemical Structure:

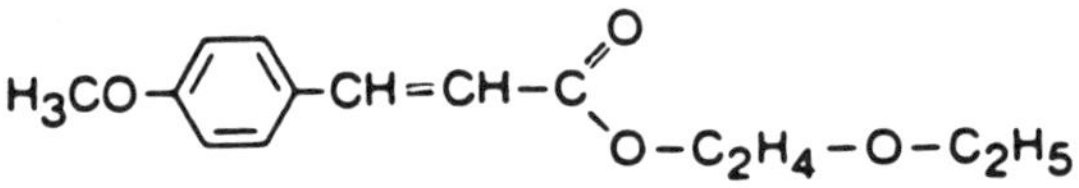

$$H_3CO-\langle\bigcirc\rangle-CH=CH-C{\overset{O}{\underset{O-C_2H_4-O-C_2H_5}{}}}$$

Synonyms: Giv Tan F

UV absorption maximum: 310nm (1)

Usual concentration: 1% to 4%

(f)

Figure 1 (cont.)

114

3-(4-methylbenzylidene)-camphor

CAS number: 36861-47-9

Chemical Structure:

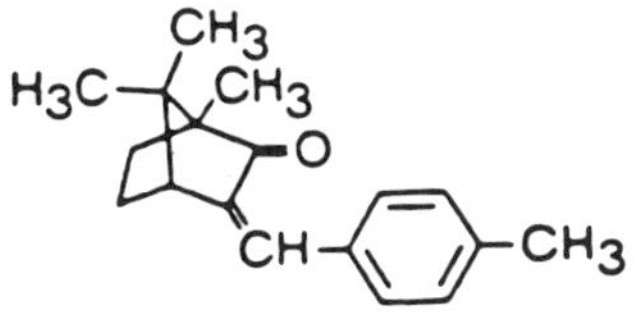

Synonyms: Eusolex 6300, 3-(4-methylbenzylidene)-2-bornanone

UV absorption maximum: 336-340nm (1,100)

Usual concentration: Up to 7.5%

(g)

Oxybenzone

CAS number: 131-57-7

Chemical Structure:

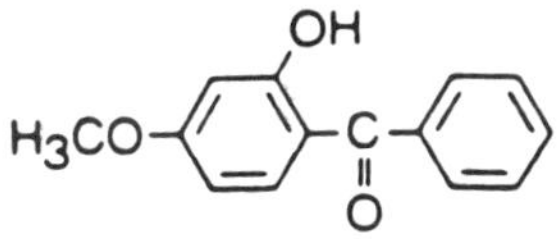

Synonyms: Eusolex 4630, (2-hydroxy-4-methoxy)-benzophenone,
(2-hydroxy-4-methoxyphenyl)-phenylmethanone

UV absorption maxima: 288-290, 325nm (1,100)

Usual concentration: 1% to 4%

(h)

Figure 1 (cont.)

incidence of side effects caused by sunscreens is about 1 to 2% with a low to medium risk index. This latter figure was based on surveys of cosmetics including the FDA pilot study (97) and the U.S. manufacturers' file (98). Of course, it could be argued that these reports, consisting mainly of single case reports, do not accurately reflect the true sensitization rates of these agents and that many mild reactions that occur in subjects may not be reported or may be interpreted as failures of sunscreen protection, as pointed out by Davies et al. (40). This is a valid criticism and the establishment of a registry for adverse reporting of sunscreening agents similar to that developed for the nonsteroidal anti-inflammatory agents by Stern and Bigby (99) would help characterize the sensitization rates of these agents. In addition, much work needs to be done not only in terms of epidemiology but in appropriate testing techniques.

REFERENCES

1. Food and Drug Administration. Sunscreen drug products for over-the-counter human drugs: proposed safety, effective and labeling conditions. *Fed. Reg., 43*:38206 (1978).
2. Horio, T. and Higuchi, T. Photocontact dermatitis from p-aminobenzoic acid. *Dermatologica, 156*:124 (1978).
3. Marmelzat, J. and Rapaport, M. J. Photodermatitis with PABA. *Contact Dermatitis, 6*:230–231 (1980).
4. Cronin, E. *Contact Dermatitis*, Churchill Livingstone, London (1980), pp. 450–454.
5. Adams, R. M., Maibach, H. I., Clendenning, W. E., et al. A five-year study of cosmetic reactions. *J. Am. Acad. Dermatol., 13*:1062 (1985).
6. Fagerlund, V-L., Kalimo, K., and Jansen, C. Valonsuoja-aineet fotokontaktiallergian aiheuttajina, *Duodecim., 99*:146 (1983).
7. Wennersten, G., Thune, P., Brodthagen, H., et al. The Scandinavian multicenter photopatch study: Preliminary results. *Contact Dermatitis, 10*:305–309 (1984).
8. Thune, P. Contact and photocontact allergy to sunscreens. *Photodermatology, 1*:5 (1984).
9. Camarasa, J. G. and Serra-Baldrich, E. Allergic contact dermatitis to sunscreens. *Contact Dermatitis, 15*:253 (1986).
10. Menz, J., Muller, S. A., and Connoly, S. M. Photopatch testing: a six-year experience. *J. Am. Acad. Dermatol., 18*:1044 (1988).
11. English, J. S. C. and White, I. R. Allergic contact dermatitis from isopropyl dibenzoylmethane. *Contact Dermatitis, 15*:94 (1986).
12. Sams, W. M. Contact photodermatitis. *Arch. Dermatol., 73*:142 (1956).
13. Pariser, R. J. Contact dermatitis to dioxybenzone. *Contact Dermatitis, 3*: 172 (1977).
14. Thompson, G., Maibach, H., and Epstein, J. Allergic contact dermatitis from sunscreen preparations complicating photodermatitis. *Arch. Dermatol., 113*:1252 (1977).

15. Baer, R. L. and Meltzer, L. Sensitization to monoglyceryl para-amino-benzoate. *J. Invest. Dermatol., 11*:5 (1948).

16. Meltzer, L. and Baer, R. L. Sensitization to monoglycerol para-amino-benzoate: a case report. *J. Invest. Dermatol., 12*:31 (1949).

17. Curtis, G. H. and Crawford, P. F. Cutaneous sensitivity to monoglycerol para-aminobenzoate. *Cleveland Clin. Q., 18*:35 (1951).

18. Goldman, G. C. and Epstein, E. Contact photosensitivity dermatitis from sun-protective agent. *Arch. Dermatol., 100*:447 (1969).

19. Fisher, A. A. Sunscreen dermatitis due to glyceryl PABA: significance of cross-reactions to this PABA ester. *Current Contact News, 18*:495 (1976).

20. Fisher, A. A. Dermatitis due to benzocaine present in sunscreens containing glyceryl PABA (Escalol 106). *Contact Dermatitis, 3*:170 (1977).

21. Caro, I. Contact allergy/photoallergy to glyceryl PABA and benzocaine. *Contact Dermatitis, 4*:381 (1978).

22. Hjorth, N., Wilkinson, D., Magnusson, B., Bandmann, H-J., and Maibach, H. Glyceryl p-aminobenzoate patch testing in benzocaine-sensitive subjects. *Contact Dermatitis, 4*:46 (1978).

23. Mathias, C. G. T., Maibach, H. I., and Epstein, J. Allergic contact photo-dermatitis to para-aminobenzoic acid. *Arch. Dermatol., 114*:1665 (1978).

24. Kroon, S. Standard photopatch testing with Waxtar, para-aminobenzoic acid, potassium chromate and balsam of Peru. *Contact Dermatitis, 18*:35 (1983).

25. Rietschel, R. L. and Lewis, C. W. Contact dermatitis to homomenthyl sali-cylate. *Arch. Dermatol., 114*:442–443 (1978).

26. Fowler, J. F. Allergic cheilitis due to benzophenone-3. Presented to the Patch Test Clinic Symposium at the American Academy of Dermatology Annual Meeting, San Antonio (1987).

27. Schauder, S. and Ippen, H. Photoallergic and allergic contact dermatitis from dibenzoylmethanes. *Photodermatology, 3*:140 (1986).

28. Schauder, S. and Ippen, H. Photoallergic and allergic contact dermatitis from dibenzoylmethane compounds and other sunscreens. *Der Hautarzt., 39*:435 (1988).

29. Ramsay, D. L., Cohen, H. J., and Baer, R. L. Allergic reaction to benzo-phenone. *Arch. Dermatol., 105*:906 (1972).

30. De Groot, A. C. and Weyland, J. W. Contact allergy to butyl methoxydi-benzoylmethane. *Contact Dermatitis, 16*:278 (1987).

31. De Groot, A. C., van der Walle, H. B., Jagtman, B. A., and Weyland, J. W. Contact allergy to 4-isopropyl-dibenzoylmethane and 3-(4-methylbenzyli-dene) camphor in sunscreen Eusolex 8021. *Contact Dermatitis, 16*:249 (1987).

32. Woods, B. Dermatitis from Eusolex 8021 sunscreen agent in a cosmetic. *Contact Dermatitis, 7*:168 (1981).

33. English, J. S. C., White, I. R., and Cronin, E. Sensitivity to sunscreens. *Contact Dermatitis, 17*:159 (1987).

34. Haussman, A. and Kleinhaus, D. Allergisches kontaktekzum durch UV-strahlenfilter in sonenschutzcremes–zwei fallbeobachtungen. *Z. Hautkr., 61*:1654 (1986).

35. Fisher, A. A. The presence of benzocaine in sunscreens containing glyceryl PABA (Escalol 106). *Arch. Dermatol., 113*:1299 (1977).
36. Millard, L. G. and Barrett, P. L. Contact allergy from Mexenone masquerading as an exacerbation of light sensitivity. *Contact Dermatitis, 3*:222 (1977).
37. Hunloh, W. and Goerz, G. Contact dermatitis from Eusolex 6300. *Contact Dermatitis, 9*:333 (1983).
38. Wennersten, G., Thune, P., Jansen, C. T., and Brodhagen, H. Photocontact dermatitis: Current status with emphasis on allergic contact photosensitivity (CPS) occurrence, allergens and practical phototesting. *Sem. Dermatol., 5*:273 (1986).
39. Goodman, T. Photodermatitis from a sunscreening agent. *Arch. Dermatol., 102*:563 (1970).
40. Davies, M. G., Hawk, J. L. M., and Rycroft, R. J. G. Acute photosensitivity from the sunscreen 2-ethoxyethyl-p-methoxycinnamate. *Contact Dermatitis, 8*:190 (1982).
41. Murphy, G. M. and White, I. R. Photoallergic contact dermatitis to ethoxyethyl-p-methoxycinnamate. *Contact Dermatitis, 16*:296 (1987).
42. Kaidbey, K. H. and Allen, H. Photocontact dermatitis to benzocaine. *Arch. Dermatol., 117*:77 (1981).
43. Holzle, E. and Plewig, G. Photoallergishe kontadermatitis durch benzophenonhaltige sonnenchutzpraparate. *Der Hautarzt., 33*:391 (1982).
44. Knobler, E., Almeida, L., Ruzkowski, A. M., Held, J., Harber, L., and DeLeo, V. Photoallergy to benzophenone. *Arch. Dermatol. 125*:801 (1989).
45. Emmett, E. A., Taphorn, B. R., and Kominsky, J. R. Phototoxicity occurring during the manufacture of ultraviolet-cured ink. *Arch. Dermatol., 113*:770 (1977).
46. Katz, S. I. Relative effectiveness of selected sunscreens. *Arch. Dermatol., 101*:466 (1970).
47. Weller, P. and Freeman, S. Photocontact allergy to octyldimethyl PABA. *Aust. J. Dermatol., 25*:73 (1984).
48. Kalimo, K., Fagerlund, V-L., and Jansen, C. Concomitant photocontact allergy to a benzophenone derivative and a sunscreen preservative, 6-acetoxy-2,4-dimethyl-m-dioxane. *Photodermatology, 1*:315 (1984).
49. Bury, J. N. Photoallergies from benzophenones and beta carotene in sunscreens. *Contact Dermatitis, 6*:211 (1980).
50. Satulsky, E. M. Photosensitization induced by monoglycerol paraaminobenzoate: a case report. *Arch. Dermatol., 62*:711 (1950).
51. Roberts, D. L. Contact allergy to Eusolex 8021. *Contact Dermatitis, 8*:302 (1988).
52. Alomar, A. and Cerda, M. T. Contact allergy to Eusolex 8021. *Contact Dermatitis, 20*:74 (1989).
53. Willis, I. Sensitization potential of para-aminobenzoic acid. *Cosmet. Toilet., 91*:63 (1976).
54. Sulzberger, M. B., Kanof, A., Baer, R. L., and Lowenberg, C. Sensitization by topical application of sulfonamides. *J. Allergy, 18*:92 (1947).

55. Bruze, M., Fregert, S., and Gruvberger, B. Occurrence of para-amino-benzoic acid and benzocaine as contaminants in sunscreen agents of para-aminobenzoic acid type. *Photodermatology, 1*:277 (1984).

56. Bruze, M., Gruvberger, B., and Thune, P. Contact and photocontact allergy to glyceryl para-aminobenzoate. *Photodermatology, 5*:162 (1988).

57. Kaidbey, K. H., and Kligman, A. M. Phototoxicity to a sunscreen in-gredient: Padimate A. *Arch. Dermatol., 114*:547 (1978).

58. Calnan, C. D. Cinnamon dermatitis from an ointment. *Contact Dermatitis, 2*:167 (1976).

59. Weyland, J. W., Rooselaar, J., Assink-Gerverinick, J. M. B., and Hartog, B. J. *Sun Cosmetics 1984*. Market Survey, Cosmetics Report No. 36. Food Inspection Service, Enschede, The Netherlands (1985).

60. Van Ketel, W. G. Allergic contact dermatitis from an aminobenzoic acid compound used in sunscreens. *Contact Dermatitis, 3*:283 (1977).

61. Mork, N-J. and Austad, J. Contact dermatitis from witisol, a sunscreen agent. *Contact Dermatitis, 10*:122 (1984).

62. Fisher, A. A. *Contact Dermatitis*, 2nd ed., Lea & Febiger, Philadelphia (1973), p. 209.

63. Kaminester, L. H. Allergic reaction to sunscreen products. *Arch. Derma-tol., 117*:66 (1981).

64. Nater, J. P. and De Groot, A. C. *Unwanted Effects of Cosmetics and Drugs Used in Dermatology*, 2nd ed., Elsevier, Amsterdam (1985), p. 360.

65. De Groot, A. C., Van der Meeren, H. L. M., and Weyland, J. W. Contact allergy to avocado oil in a sunscreen. *Contact Dermatitis, 16*:108 (1987).

66. Edwards, E. K. and Edwards, E. K. Allergic reaction to t-butyl alcohol in a sunscreen. *Cutis, 29*:476 (1982).

67. Edwards, E. K. and Edwards, E. K. Allergic reaction of triethanolamine stearate. *Cutis, 31*:195 (1983).

68. Edwards, E. K. Allergic reactions to benzyl alcohol in a sunscreen. *Cutis, 28*:332 (1981).

69. Hannuksela, M. Skin contact allergy to emulsifiers. *Int. J. Cosmetic Sci., 10*:9 (1988).

70. De Groot, A. C. and Weyland, J. W. Hidden contact allergy to formalde-hyde in imidazolidinyl urea. *Contact Dermatitis, 17*:124 (1987).

71. Dooms-Goossens, A., De Boulle, K., Doom, M., and De Groot, H. Imidazo-lidinyl urea dermatitis. *Contact Dermatitis, 1*:322 (1986).

72. Methylisothiazolinone additional skin retention data. *Rose Sheet*, April 25, 1988, p. 7.

73. Ford, G. P. and Beck, M. H. Reactions to quarternium 15, bronopol and Germall 115 in a standard series. *Contact Dermatitis, 14*:271 (1986).

74. De Groot, A. C., Bruynzeel, D. P., Bos, J. D., et al. The allergens in cosmetics. *Arch. Dermatol., 124*:1525 (1988).

75. De Groot, A. C., Weyland, J. W., Bos, J. D., and Jagtman, B. A. Contact allergy to preservatives (I). *Contact Dermatitis, 14*:120 (1986).

76. Hannuksela, M., Kousa, M., and Pirila, V. Allergy ingredients of vehicles. *Contact Dermatitis, 2*:105 (1976).

77. Fransway, A. F. Sensitivity to Kathon CG: findings in 365 consecutive patients. *Contact Dermatitis, 19*:342 (1988).
78. Baer, R. L. Cross-sensitization phenomenon, *Modern Trends in Dermatology* (R. M. B. McKenna, ed.), Butterworths, London (1954), p. 232.
79. Dupuis, G. and Benezra, C. Cross-sensitization, *Allergic Contact Dermatitis to Simple Chemicals. A Molecular Approach*, Marcel Dekker, Inc., New York (1982), pp. 87–126.
80. MacLeod, T. M. and Frain-Bell, W. The study of the efficacy of some agents used for the protection of the skin from exposure to light. *Br. J. Dermatol., 84*:266 (1971).
81. Thune, P. and Eeg-Larsen, T. Contact and photocontact allergy in persistent light reactivity. *Contact Dermatitis, 11*:98 (1984).
82. Addo, H. A. and Frain-Bell, W. Persistence of allergic contact sensitivity in subjects with photosensitivity dermatitis and actinic reticuloid syndrome. *Br. J. Dermatol., 117*:555 (1987).
83. Addo, H. H. A., Sharma, S. C., Ferguson, J., et al. A study of composite plant extract reactions in photosensitivity dermatitis. *Photodermatology, 2*:68 (1985).
84. Fisher, A. A. The role of nonsensitizing alternatives in the management of allergic contact dermatitis. *Sem. Dermatol., 5*:263 (1986).
85. Bruze, M., Fregert, S., and Luggren, B. Effect of ultraviolet irradiation of photopatch test substances in vitro. *Photodermatology, 2*:32 (1985).
86. Epstein, S. Masked photopatch tests. *Contact Dermatitis, 41*:369 (1963).
87. Maibach, H. I., Akerson, J. M., Marzulli, F. N., et al. Test concentrations and vehicles for dermatological testing of cosmetic ingredients. *Contact Dermatitis, 6*:369 (1980).
88. Fischer, T., and Maibach, H. I. Patch testing in allergic contact dermatitis: An update. *Sem. Dermatol., 5*:214 (1980).
89. Rycroft, R. J. G. False reactions to non-standard patch tests. *Sem. Dermatol., 5*:225 (1986).
90. Bruynzeel, D. P. and Maibach, H. I. Excited skin syndrome (angry back). *Arch. Dermatol., 122*:323 (1986).
91. Parrish, J. A., Pathak, M. A., and Fitzpatrick, T. B. Facial irritation due to sunscreen products. *Arch. Dermatol., 111*:525 (1975).
92. Calnan, C. D. Stinging sensation from ethoxyethyl-methoxy cinnamate. *Contact Dermatitis, 4*:294 (1978).
93. Cullen, S. I. Safety and efficacy of two sunscreens in tretinoin-treated acne vulgaris. *Curr. Ther. Res., 26*:625 (1979).
94. Forbes, M. A., Brannen, M., and King, W. C. Benzophenone as a sunscreen. *South. Med. J., 59*:321 (1966).
95. Von Krogh, G. and Maibach, H. I. The contact urticaria syndrome, *Dermatotoxicology*, 3rd ed. (F. N. Marzulli and H. I. Maibach, eds.), Hemisphere Publishing Company, Washington, DC, Chap. 15.
96. Lammintansta, K., Maibach, H. I., and Wilson, D. Mechanisms of subjective (sensory) irritation. Propensity to non-immunologic contact urticaria and objective irritation in stingers. *Derm. Beruf. Umwelt., 36*:45 (1988).

97. *(PB-242 480) An investigation of Consumers' perception of adverse reactions to cosmetic products.* (1975). Westat Inc., prepared for the Food and Drug Administration, National Technical Information Service U.S. Department of Commerce, Springfield, Virginia.
98. *Tabulation of Cosmetic Product Experience Report, Submitted to the Food and Drug Administration under Voluntary Cosmetic Regulatory Program (Jan 1974–June 1975),* Food and Drug Administration, Division of Cosmetic Technology, Washington, DC.
99. Stern, R. S. and Bigby, M. An expanded profile of cutaneous reactions to nonsteroidal anti-inflammatory drugs, Reports to a specialty-based system for spontaneous reporting of adverse reactions to drugs. *JAMA 252*: 1433 (1984).
100. Shaath, N. A. Encyclopedia of UV absorbers for sunscreen products. *Cosmet. Toilet., 102*:21 (1987).

NOTE ADDED IN PROOF

After submission of the original manuscript, there have been several additional reports of photosensitization/sensitization to sunscreening agents, including two cases of contact allergy to bornelone (de Groot and Weyland); two cases of contact allergy to isopropyldibenzoylmethane (Garioch and Forsyth) and one case of photocontact allergy to a sunscreen containing isopropyldibenzoylmethane and 3-(4'-methylbenzylidene) camphor (Foussereau, Cavelier, and Protois); one case of photocontact allergy to isopropyldibenzoylmethane and *t*-butyl methoxy dibenzoylmethane (Motley and Reynolds) and four cases of photocontact allergy to oxybenzone (Marguery and Bazex). In addition to these case reports, the final report of the five-year Scandinavian multicenter photopatch study was published (Thune et al. 1988). The report included 33 cases of contact and photocontact allergy to the following sunscreening agents; *p*-aminobenzoic acid (14), glyceryl PABA (3), padimate A (3), padimate O (5), cinoxate (3), 2-phenylbenzimidazole-5-sulfonic acid (2), isopropyl-methoxy-dibenzoylmethane (1), and 3-(4-methyl-benzylidene camphor (2). These reports are not included in Table 1.

REFERENCES ADDED IN PROOF

de Groot, A. C. and Weyland, J. W. Cosmetic allergy to the UV-absorber bornelone. *Dermatosen., 37*:13 (1989).
Foussereau, J., Cavelier, C. and Protois, J. C. Contact dermatitis from Eusolex 8021 elucidated by chemical analysis. *Contact Dermatitis, 20*:311 (1989).
Garioch, J. J. and Forsyth, A. Allergic contact dermatitis from 4-isopropyl-dibenzoylmethane in a light moisturising cream. *Contact Dermatitis, 20*:312 (1989).

Marguery, M. C. and Bazex, J. Photocontact dermatitis due to 2-hydroxy, 4-methoxybenzophenone (oxybenzone): report of four cases. *Brit. J. Dermatol., Suppl. 34, 121*:59 (1989).

Motley, R. J. and Reynolds, A. J. Photocontact dermatitis due to isopropyl and butyl methoxy dibenzoylmethanes (Eusolex 8020 and Parsol 1789). *Contact Dermatitis, 21*:109 (1989).

9
Sunscreens and Hair

SERGIO NACHT *Advanced Polymer Systems Inc., Redwood City, California*

Throughout the history of the development of sun protection, little attention has been given to the use of sunscreens on hair. This lack of interest is most likely due to the fact that hair does not develop cancer or wrinkle with age like its parent tissue, the skin. Nor does this skin appendage burn or become very uncomfortable from too much sun exposure.

Yet men and women through the centuries have experienced noticeable changes in the properties of their hair after exposure to ultraviolet radiation. Today, one can still find field workers wearing hats as they toil in the sun, and hair-conscious sunbathers will frequently don a scarf before seeking the sun's rays. These people have discovered that sunlight does produce undesirable changes in hair quality. Dryness, reduced strength, rough surface texture, loss of color and luster, stiffness and brittleness have been reported by both the lay population and the research community (1-7), although only a sparse collection of quantitative data regarding the effects of ultraviolet light to human hair is available.

When absorbed, ultraviolet radiation is responsible for the photochemical degradation of many substances within the skin (8-11). Sunscreens have been proven to reduce the chemical effects of ultraviolet light to the skin (12-15) and have become popular with consumers during the past decade. To determine the protective efficacy of topical sunscreen products, a sun protection factor (SPF) scale was proposed by the OTC-FDA Advisory Review Panel in their proposed monograph addressing sunscreens as over the counter (OTC) drugs in 1978 (6). However, no mention is made in this monograph concerning sunscreen efficacy on hair protein.

In this chapter, we discuss some of the photochemical changes occurring in hair, the effects that sunscreens have on reducing these changes, and we propose a method and a numerical scale for the determination of sunscreen efficacy for hair protection which we labeled the hair protection factor (HPF).

I. MECHANISMS OF HAIR WEATHERING

Hair is the recipient of a constant series of environmental assaults we term "weathering." Such potentially damaging influences as rain, air pollutants, wind, sea water, or chemicals in swimming pools contribute to the environmental processes known to cause structural and chemical degradation to hair (2).

Most damaging of all environmental factors is ultraviolet radiation (1–3). These effects are compounded when combined with other environmentally and chemically induced damage (as in the cases of hair bleaches, colorants, and permanent wave products) (2).

An example of this damage is the condition of a cuticle on a normal unexposed hair as compared with a cuticle covering hair that has been exposed to ultraviolet radiation, either singularly or in association with other elements. The cuticle is considered to play a key role in determining the overall physical properties in keratin fibers (3), whereas the interior of the fiber, the cortex, is believed to have less importance with respect to hair condition (1). The cuticle dictates the frictional properties of the hair fibers and is also largely responsible for the integrity of the interior. In normal hair, defined as hair that has not been exposed to the environment or chemical processing, the edges of the cuticle cells are smooth, rounded and tightly packed onto the cortex. Long-term exposure of hair to sunlight and the atmosphere results in the breakdown of cuticle cells on the hair surface (1). Thus, cleavage of the cuticle cells coating exposed hair have been observed within the endocuticle layer of these hairs in many instances (3). This results in the alteration of the mechanical properties of human hair.

II. ULTRAVIOLET RADIATION AND CHEMICAL DEGRADATION OF HAIR

Several photochemical reactions occur in hair after exposure to ultraviolet radiation. Discoloration, often called "highlights" observed by sunbathers the world over, is the most obvious chemical alteration caused by the sun. But other, subtler chemical changes occur that are evident to the human eye only after they have accumulated over time or by the intensity of exposure.

A. Discoloration

Fading of brown hair and yellowing of blond and red hair have been observed by several researchers (6, 17). The fading of brown hair is attributed to be a result of the photooxidative bleaching of melanin hair pigment (2), while discoloration of blond hair has been explained in terms of the photodegradation of cystine, tyrosine, and tryptophan residues, producing yellowing and brown reaction products (18-21). Degradation of histidine, lysine, and proline have also been discovered (2) and are thought to be responsible for some of the yellow discolorations of blond hair (6).

Pheomelanin, predominant in red and blond shades, is also present in brown hair, which appears to be a mixture of this lighter melanin pigment and the darker eumelanin. Eumelanin is chemically different from pheomelanin, the most obvious difference being the higher sulfur content of the lighter pigment compared to that of eumelanin (22). It has been reported that superoxides are formed when pheomelanin is degraded by irradiation with long-wavelength ultraviolet and visible light (23-26). This sensitivity of pheomelanin can explain why the most obvious discolorations occur in lighter hair shades, while becoming less apparent in darker tones of hair containing higher levels of eumelanin.

B. Sorption Characteristics

Changes in the sorption characteristics and urea/bisulfite solubility of hair have been detected upon extended weathering exposure (2,6,27). The increase in urea/bisulfite solubility suggests that a network of new types of crosslinks are formed during the weathering process, especially as it relates to ultraviolet radiation (27). Although not much is known about the exact chemical structure of these crosslinks, several isopeptides which are not present in intact hair were found in enzymic hydrolysates of weathered fibers (2,27,28).

C. The Free Radical Mechanism

Recently, a free radical mechanism has been proposed which may account for many of the photochemical changes occurring in weathered human hair (2,27, 29). Ultraviolet radiation is absorbed by cystine, tyrosine, phenylalanine, and tryptophan residues, and possibly some peptide bonds, which results in the formation of free radicals. Homolytic scission of disulfide bonds then occurs.

In the presence of such free radical carriers as water, present as humidity in the atmosphere, a sequence of radical transfer reactions involving hydroxyl radicals can take place. This causes random displacements along the protein backbone that leads to an assortment of degradation products (2).

Free radical formation appears to be affected by melanin, which is believed to act as an energy "sink" (29), thus protecting keratin against radiation in the initial stages of weathering. Heavily pigmented hair has a high absorption capacity that is explained in terms of its comprehensive system of double bonds and conjugated carbonyl groups (2). Large fractions of ultraviolet light may be captured by the melanin via this absorption process, which also immobilizes free radicals as they are formed. This activity prevents the propagation of free radicals into underlying keratin structures.

D. Tensile Strength

Tensile strength of hair fibers has been shown to decrease in correlation to ultraviolet radiation exposure time (2,6,17,30). Reduced cystine levels accompanied by the generation of cysteic acid are found in hair exposed to the environment, resulting in the destruction of stabilizing disulfide bonds (2,27–29,31). Pigmented fibers exhibit less cystine reduction than those that are nonpigmented (2). This reduction appears to be unrelated to the level of humidity present during exposure.

While pronounced tensile alteration is due primarily to photochemical effects on disulfide linkages (30), deamination, or decarboxylation of amino acids (32), disorientation of hydrogen bonds and the chemical alteration of the aromatic nuclei in tyrosine and phenylalanine (33) also contribute to a chemical reduction in tensile strength.

Another factor influencing the correlation of hair tensile strength to ultraviolet exposure is seasonal radiation. Summer solar radiation has been found to be five times greater than that received by hair during the winter months (31).

III. SUNSCREENS AND HAIR PROTECTION

Because of the obvious photochemical degradation of hair, several researchers have suggested the use of some form of chemical protection from the sun (2,8, 17). Although many sunscreens are available for use in skin protection, only a few lend themselves to use in hair care products.

The ideal sunscreen for hair must be substantive to the hair cuticle even in the presence of surfactants, without causing loss of sheen or adding a "gummy" quality to hair. Yet this sunscreen must also be easily incorporated into the largely water-based vehicles used on the hair by consumers. Few sunscreens possess these qualitites while maintaining the water-resistance required for long-term hair protection. In a variety of tests (17), octyl-dimethyl PABA was found to be the most suitable of all sunscreens recognized in the OTC-FDA sunscreen monograph (16) while para amino benzoic acid (PABA) is the least desirable due to its high water solubility and low substantivity to hair.

IV. ASSESSING PROTECTIVE EFFICACY OF SUNSCREENS
FOR HAIR

As sunscreen protection becomes an accepted practice in hair care, a simple yet accurate technique is needed to assess protective efficacy of sunscreen ingredients and formulations designed for hair use. A parametric scale for the comparison of the performance of these sunscreen products on the hair is also required.

A. Sun Protection Factor

To determine the protective efficacy of sunscreen products applied to the skin, a sun protection factor (SPF) scale was proposed by the OTC-FDA Advisory Review Panel in their monograph addressing sunscreens (16). This scale provides consumers with a simple numerical identification of the different levels of protection offered by various commercial products.

The SPF is defined as the ratio of the ultraviolet energy required to produce minimal erythema on protected skin to that required to produce the same minimal erythema on unprotected skin in the same individual.

To ensure reproducibility and provide a meaningful comparison between products, the OTC-FDA panel recommended specific testing procedures that are now followed by most manufacturers of sunscreen products to determine the SPF ratings of their products.

B. Hair Protection Factor

The SPF scale is directly related to a perceivable change in the skin, notably sunburn. Hair damage due to ultraviolet radiation does not result in a change so easily perceived by either the consumer or the researcher. Therefore, a scale which accurately measures hair damage and determines the protective effects of hair treatments containing sunscreens must use a different end-point than that used for skin. This scale could be termed the hair protection factor (HPF).

A practical HPF can be determined by measuring the ultraviolet damage to hair as detected by yield slope analysis of tensile strength assessments (17,30). When hair is extended with a tensile strength tester, the changes in the slope of the stress-strain curve in the yield region correlate well with the amount of ultraviolet radiation to which the hair has been exposed. Then, when the negative, inverse logarithm of the yield slope ($-1/\ln$) is plotted versus exposure time, a straight line is obtained between 0 and 3 hours.

Since consumers have been educated, primarily by industry, to understand an SPF scale which basically ranges from 2 through 15, we have chosen to arbitrarily construct a similar scale to facilitate the analogy. Therefore, to construct the HPF scale, the line obtained with a sample of virgin, untreated hair is arbitrarily divided into 15 divisions, with "0" set at the 3 hour point for maximum damage, and "15" located at the no exposure value for no ultraviolet damage.

A perfect analogy with the SPF scale used for skin protection would have come from a definition such as:

$$HPF = \frac{\text{(yield slope, nonirradiated} - \text{yield slope, irradiated) unprotected hair}}{\text{(yield slope, nonirradiated} - \text{yield slope, irradiated) protected hair}}$$

However, simple calculations of protection factors with such an equation using the yield slope values obtained in our experiments result in an "unnatural" scale which provides exceedingly small numbers at the lower end of the scale, while resulting in very large numbers (that tend to infinity as the denominator gets smaller) when the treatment provides good protection. These distortions make such a scale impractical and probably difficult for the consumer to understand since it could easily yield numbers as large as 200.

For this reason we have chosen to utilize the seemingly more convoluted, but more practical, logarithmic scale above stated.

V. METHODOLOGY FOR DETERMINING HPF

A. Hair Tensile Strength As a Measurement of HPF

Hair passes through three phases while being extended under increasing force (Fig. 1). The first phase, the elastic region, is characterized by reversible extension. Hydrogen bonds are probably the only ones disturbed in this region. The

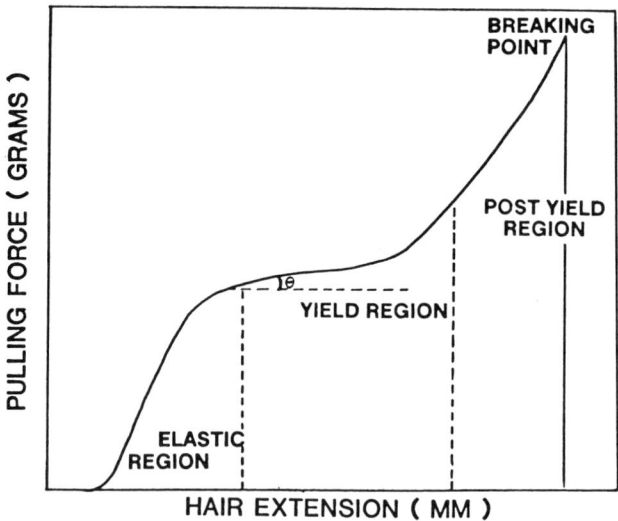

Figure 1   Typical stress-strain curve of a single hair fiber as obtained with an Instrom tensile strength tester.

second phase is characterized by a partially reversible transformation in which covalent and salt bonds are likely to be disturbed. This phase is known as the yield region. Leading to the breaking point is the post yield region, or third phase. This is where complete fiber breakage occurs.

Other research (34) has shown that the breaking point of hair is related to hair diameter, and may not necessarily be an indication of overall hair damage. Therefore, this parameter seems not to be accurate or sensitive enough to measure subtle degrees of hair damage.

Since the yield region is the one most likely to correlate in general with covalent and possibly with disulfide bond breakage in hair, and since these are the types of bonds most probably affected by ultraviolet radiation which results in intrinsic structural hair damage, evaluation of the yield slope can provide a practical and objective measurement of hair damage due to ultraviolet exposure.

B. Determination of Hair Tensile Strength

Hair tensile strength is determined by positioning a single strand of hair, about 30 cm long, between the two clamps of an Instron tensile strength tester (35) set at a standardized distance of 23 cm. The hair is then pulled with a 20 g load setting at a crosshead speed of 100 mm/min and at a chart speed of 200 mm/min. All measurements are made in an environmental chamber set at 22°C and 20% relative humidity (RH). At least 20 single hair strands from each group are extended. From the stress-strain graphs obtained for each hair, the slope of the yield region (Fig. 1) is measured and averaged for the group.

It is apparent that the differences in cross-sectional area of the hair can affect the accuracy of the yield-slope determination (Table 1). However, using a trained technician to pick hair of average size and similar cross-sectional area, it is possible to reproducibly select hair of average diameter.

Table 1 Assessment of Different Hair Diameter by Yield Slope Analysis

		Average yield slope + SD[a]
Virgin untreated 30–50 units DIA	N = 20	0.159 ± 0.053
Virgin untreated 60–80 units DIA	N = 20	0.287 ± 0.103
Virgin untreated random sample[b] 30–80 units DIA	N = 40	0.230 ± 0.075

[a]Standard deviation.
[b]Average size hair randomly selected by the trained technician.

C. Determination of Sun-Induced Damage to Hair

Virgin hair at least 30 cm long is spread apart in a single layer and uniformly exposed for different lengths of time to a Kratos solar simulator (36) adjusted to 20 volts and 30 amperes at a fixed distance of 64 cm. The solar simulator suggested for use in these tests provides a highly intensified spectrum of light which closely resembles solar radiation and, thus, is capable of accelerating the damage to hair produced by sun exposure. Although a small increase in temperature may be observed after extensive exposure with the solar simulator, this increase in temperature has been found to have no effect in the yield slope of hair (17).

After various times of exposure, the stress-strain curve of hair is determined as previously described. The mean yield slope for the 20 single hair strands in each group of ultraviolet exposed hair is then calculated as indicated above. These results can be compared to the mean yield slope of a similar group of virgin (untreated, unexposed) hair representing the value for totally undamaged hair.

D. Evaluation of HPF

Swatches of hair in excess of 20 strands, are prepared from the same sample of virgin hair as that used for standardization. These swatches are soaked for 30 minutes in the test solution and rinsed for 30 seconds with warm tap water (37°C). This procedure is repeated four times. Although this soaking cycle may seem exaggerated, results are produced that are similar to those obtained from 20 cycles of two minute soakings in a shampoo followed by rinsing (17). This regimen reflects accelerated one month in vivo usage conditions (Table 2). Consequently, the four-cycle regimen is recommended for simplicity. For leave-on

Table 2 Effect of Treatment Regimen on HPF Value

Treatment[a]	Regimen	Yield slope + SD	HPF (0–15)
0.2% Octyl-dimethyl PABA	4 cycles 30' per cycle	0.309 ± 0.073	6.6
0.2% Octyl-dimethyl PABA	20 cycles 2' per cycle	0.313 ± 0.066	7.1
0.5% Octyl-dimethyl PABA	4 cycles 30' per cycle	0.346 ± 0.057	11.6
0.5% Octyl-dimethyl PABA	20 cycles 2' per cycle	0.348 ± 0.055	11.9

[a]All treatments consisted of a commercial shampoo (Pantene Shampoo for Normal Hair) containing various concentration of octyl-dimethyl para amino benzoic acid.

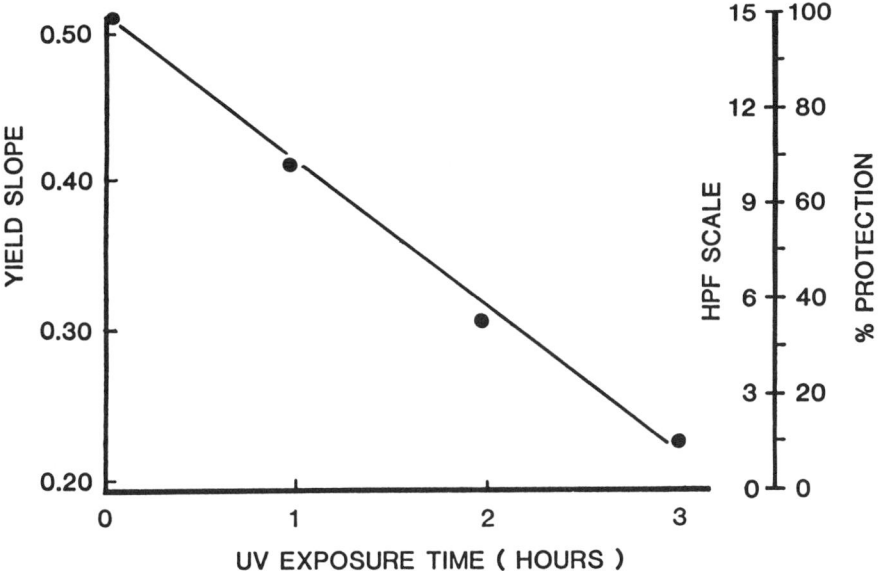

Figure 2 Decrease in yield slope with increased exposure of hair to UV radiation. Definition of the hair protection factor (HPF) scale.

products, such as hair sprays and mousses, the hair swatches are treated four times with the products as directed for use. After treatment by either shampoo or leave-on products, the hair swatches are air-dried overnight at room temperature.

These treated swatches are then exposed to the solar simulator for 3 hours, as previously described. After exposure, hair strands are tested with the tensile strength tester and the mean yield slope is calculated for each treatment group.

The HPF provided by the product undergoing testing can now be determined by calculating the mean yield slope obtained with the exposed, treated hair and interpolating that value in the standard curve determined with untreated samples of the same hair (Fig. 2).

VI. FACTORS INFLUENCING HPF

Various factors can influence the results obtained using the suggested methodology to determine HPF.

A. Sunscreen Concentration

When tested in a simple shampoo (37), the level of protection provided by the shampoo treatment rises with the increase in sunscreen concentration (Table 3)

Table 3   Effect of Sunscreen Concentration on HPF

Treatment	Yield slope + SD	HPF
Simple shampoo[a]	0.296 ± 0.061	0.4
0.2% Octyl-dimethyl PABA in simple shampoo	0.319 ± 0.033	2.3
0.5% Octyl-dimethyl PABA in simple shampoo	0.380 ± 0.059	7.1
1.0% Octyl-dimethyl PABA in simple shampoo	0.410 ± 0.041	9.8

[a]Shampoo consisting of sodium lauryl ether sulfate and citric acid.

(17). Thus, using a scale where 15 represents total hair protection, one percent octyl-dimethyl PABA results in an HPF of 9.8, while a 0.2% concentration of this same sunscreen in the same shampoo provides an HPF of 2.3. This value can be no different from that offered by a commercial shampoo without sunscreen (Table 4). Therefore, 0.2% of octyl-dimethyl PABA may not be sufficient to provide measurable sun protection benefits to hair.

B. Shampoo Composition

Other ingredients frequently used in hair care products may enhance or reduce the spreadability and substantivity of the sunscreen and may therefore influence the sun protection ability of the total formulation. To determine these effects,

Table 4   Hair Protection Factor (HPF) of Various Concentrations of Octyl-Dimethyl-PABA in a Commercial Shampoo

Treatment	Yield slope + SD	HPF
Commercial shampoo[a]	0.321 ± 0.032	2.7
0.1% Sunscreen in commercial shampoo	0.354 ± 0.036	4.7
0.2% Sunscreen in commercial shampoo	0.391 ± 0.045	8.7
0.5% Sunscreen in commercial shampoo	0.438 ± 0.043	12.8
0.7% Sunscreen in commercial shampoo	0.417 ± 0.037	11.0

[a]As in Table 2.

Table 5   Hair Protection Factor (HPF) of Various Commercial Shampoos

Treatment	HPF
Johnson's baby shampoo	1.5
Mill Creek henna shampoo (PABA)[a]	2.7
Silkience shampoo	3.0
Pioneer brand jojoba shampoo (PABA)[a]	3.9

[a]Type of sunscreen as identified in ingredients listing.

the HPF of a commercial shampoo containing different levels of sunscreen were evaluated. The data (Tables 4 and 5) show that, at various levels of sunscreen concentration, a higher HPF is obtained with a commercial shampoo containing conditioners than those previously attained with a simple shampoo formula (17).

These results suggest that the conditioning ingredients found in many hair care formulations can enhance sunscreen protection of hair, perhaps by enhancing sunscreen substantivity or by promoting even distribution of the sunscreen over the entire hair strand.

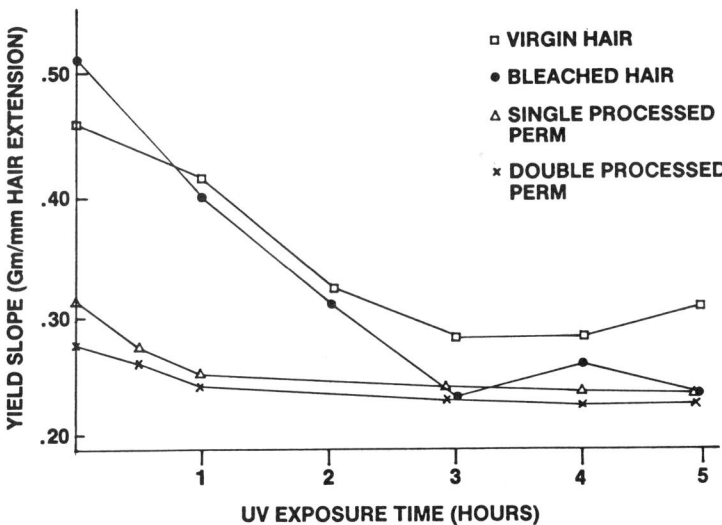

Figure 3   Comparison of the damage induced on different types of hair by increasing exposure to UV radiation.

Table 6 Effects of Sunscreen Concentration on HPF[a]

Treatment	Yield slope			HPF		
	Virgin	Bleached	Permed	Virgin	Bleached	Permed
Base shampoo	0.189 ± 0.057	0.195 ± 0.053	0.178 ± 0.041	0	0	0
0.2% Octyl-dimethyl PABA in base shampoo	0.200 ± 0.052	0.200 ± 0.057	0.176 ± 0.042	4.0	4.0	0
0.5% Octyl-dimethyl PABA in base shampoo	0.204 ± 0.056	0.204 ± 0.046	0.180 ± 0.046	5.4	5.4	2.0
1.0% Octyl-dimethyl PABA in base shampoo	0.216 ± 0.060	0.210 ± 0.058	0.184 ± 0.051	9.6	10.7	6.6

[a]Different hair samples were used.

C. Hair Type and Cosmetic History

Ultraviolet exposure of chemically processed hair increases the damage already present, frequently resulting in the maximum damage which can be produced to hair. Maximum damage for both virgin and bleached hair is achieved after 3 hours of ultraviolet exposure to the solar simulator (Fig. 3). Interestingly, HPF values obtained using treatments with increasing percentages of sunscreen are similar between virgin and bleached hair (Table 6). This similarity in the correlation of ultraviolet exposure and hair damage observed with both groups, suggests that ultraviolet radiation disrupts covalent bonds at a similar rate in both of these hair types.

On the other hand, maximum damage induced by ultraviolet radiation in permed hair occurs within less than one hour of exposure (Fig. 3). The waving solution of a permanent wave product reduces the disulfide bonds, but not all of those bonds are reformed during the neutralization phase. Therefore, permed hair is already severely damaged prior to ultraviolet exposure and suffers maximal damage much more quickly than other types of hair.

HPF can therefore be determined with virgin or bleached hair with good precision and reproducibility, but the use of severely damaged hair is not recommended.

VII. HPF AND THE FUTURE OF SUNSCREENS FOR HAIR PROTECTION

As outlined in this chapter, the hair protection factor has several major attributes in determining sunscreen protection in a broad spectrum of products.

1. HPF, as it is defined here, can be easily determined for a variety of hair types
2. A variety of formulations and sunscreen ingredients may be tested accurately using this scale
3. Unlike SPF, which is based on minimal erythemal dose and therefore responds only to UVB exposure, HPF reflects the effects of all segments of the ultraviolet spectrum
4. Since the proposed HPF scale is based on the assessment of changes in the mechanical properties of hair which are a reflection of the breakage of various keratin bonds, this scale can be of value in determining also the effects of other non-sunscreen components that may help repair or reform these bonds (i.e., free radical scavengers, disulfide bond repairers, etc.)

Finally, as the effects of sunlight on hair are better understood and appreciated by both the consumer and research communities, sunscreens are becoming an accepted ingredient in many hair care formulations. Sunscreens are especially appropriate for the protection of hair that is already perceived by the consumer as being damaged, as in weathered or chemically processed hair. While shampoos and conditioners are the obvious vehicles for such products, hair sprays, styling gels, mousses and other styling aids can also be considered for sunscreen additions.

REFERENCES

1. Breuer, M. M., Gikas, G. X., and Smith, I. T. Physical chemistry of hair condition. *Cosmet. Toilet., 94*:29–34 (1979).
2. Tolgyesi, E. Weathering of hair. *Cosmet. Toilet., 98*:29-33 (1983).
3. Hunter, L. D., Garcia, M. L., Newman, W., and Cohen, G. L. Observation of the internal structure of the human hair cuticle cell by SEM. *Text. Res. J.,* 136–140 (1974).
4. Berth, P. and Reese, G. Alteration of hair keratin by cosmetic processing and natural environmental influences. *J. Soc. Cosmet. Chem., 15*:659–666 (1964).
5. Rook, A. The clinical importance of "weathering" in human hair. *Br. J. Dermatol., 95*:111 (1976).
6. Tolgyesi, E., Peloquin, L., and Arnold, G. B. Unpublished results of an investigation conducted at Gilette Research Institute, Rockville, MD (1980).
7. Robbins, C. Weathering in human hair. *Text. Res. J., 37*:337 (1967).
8. Strobel, A. and Inserra, J. J. The use of UV absorbers in cosmetic products. *Am. Perf. Cosmet., 83*:25–30 (1968).
9. Kligman, L. H. and Kligman, A. M. The nature of photoaging: Its preventation and repair. *Photodermatology, 3*:215–227 (1986).
10. Hersey, P., MacDonald, M., Henderson, C., Schibeci, S., D'Alessandro, G., Pryor, M., and Wilkinson, F. Suppression of natural killer cell activity in humans by radiation from solarium lamps depleted of UVB. *J. Invest. Dermatol., 90*:305–310 (1988).
11. Cleaver, J. DNA damage and repair in light-sensitive human skin. *J. Invest. Dermatol., 54*:181–195 (1970).
12. Pathak, M. A. Sunscreens: topical and systemic approaches for protection of human skin against harmful effects of solar radiation. *J. Am. Acad. Dermatol., 7*:285–312 (1982).
13. Fitzpatrick, T. B., Pathak, M. A., Harber, L. C., Seiji, M., and Kukita, A. *Sunlight and Man*, University of Tokyo Press, Tokyo (1974).
14. Grove, G. L. and Kaidbey, K. H. Sunscreens prevent sunburn cell formation in human skin. *J. Invest. Dermatol., 75*:363-364 (1980).
15. Hersey, P., MacDonald, M., Burns, C., Schibeci, S., Matthews, H., and Wilkinson, F. Analysis of the effect of a sunscreen agent on the suppression of natural killer cell activity induced in human subjects by radiation from solarium lamps. *J. Invest. Dermatol., 88*:271-275 (1900).
16. FDA: Sunscreen drug product for over-the-counter human drugs; Proposed Rules, part II. *Federal Register*, 38206 (1978).

17. Nacht, S., Yeung, D., and Dunn, L. Unpublished results of an investigation conducted at Richardson-Vicks Inc., Shelton, CT (1982).
18. Speakman, J. B. and MacMahan, P. R. The action of light on wool and related fibers. *N.Z.J. Sci. Technol., 20*:2488 (1939).
19. Lennox, F. G. A spectrophotometric study of yellowing in wool fabric. *J. Text. Inst., 51*:1193 (1960).
20. Milligan, B. and Tucker, D. J. Studies on wool yellowing, Part III: Sunlight yellowing. *Text. Res. J., 33*:773 (1963).
21. Holt, L. A. and Milligan, B. The involvement of tryptophan in the photo-yellowing of wool. *J. Text. Inst., 67*:269 (1976).
22. Menon, I. A., Surujdeen, P., Haberman, H. F., and Kurian, C. J. A comparative study of the physical and chemical properties of melanins isolated from human black and red hair. *J. Invest. Dermatol., 80*:202–206 (1983).
23. Chedekel, M. R., Post, P. W., Deibel, R. M., and Kalus, M. Photodestruction of phaeomelanin. *Photochem. Photobiol., 26*:651–653 (1977).
24. Chedekel, M. R., Smith, S. K., Post, P. W., Pokora, A., and Vessell, D. L. Photodestruction of phaeomelanin: role of oxygen. *Proc. Natl. Acad. Sci. (USA), 75*:5395–5399 (1978).
25. Agin, P. R., Sayre, R. M., and Chedekel, M. R. Photodegradation of phaeomelanin: an in vitro model. *Photochem. Photobiol., 31*:359–362 (1980).
26. Chedekel, M. R., Agin, P. P., and Sayre, R. M. Photochemistry of phaeomelanin: action spectrum for superoxide production. *Photochem. Photobiol., 31*:553–555 (1980).
27. Wolfram, L. J. The reactivity of human hair, *A Review in Hair Research Status and Future Aspects* (C. E. Orfanos, W. Montagna, and G. Stuttgen, eds.), Springer-Verlog, Berlin (1981), p. 479.
28. Wolfram, L. J. Unpublished results of an investigation carried out at CSIRO, Melbourne, Australia (1973).
29. Scott, E. and Wolfram, L. J. The weathering of pigmented hair. Proc. 4th Int. Wool Text. Res. Conf., Berkeley, 1970.
30. Beyak, R., Kass, G. S., and Meyer, C. F. Elasticity and tensile properties of human hair, II. Light radiation effects. *J. Soc. Cosmet. Chem., 22*:667–687 (1971).
31. Robbins, C. R. and Kelly, C. H. Amino acid composition of human hair. *Text. Res. J., 40*:89 (1970).
32. Luse, R. A. and McLaren, A. D. Mechanism of enzyme inactivation by ultraviolet light and the photochemistry of amino acids. *Photochem. Photobiol., 2*:343–360 (1963).
33. Alexander, P. and Lett, J. T. Effects of ionizing radiations on biological macromolecules. *Comp. Biochem., 27*:157–209 (1967).
34. Collins, J. D. and Chaikin, M. The stress-strain behaviour of dimensionally and structurally, non-uniform wool fibers in water. *Text. Res. J., 35*:777–787 (1965).
35. Instron, Model #1122.
36. Kratos Solar Simulator, Model #LH153.

IV
BIOLOGICAL EVALUATION
OF SUNSCREEN PRODUCTS

10

Intrinsic and Extrinsic Photoprotection Against UVB and UVA Radiation

LEONARD C. HARBER, VINCENT A. DeLEO, and JANET H. PRYSTOWSKY
College of Physicians and Surgeons of Columbia University, New York, New York

Numerous factors serve to protect against ultraviolet (UV) radiation, including endogenous components of the skin, exogenous physical barriers, and pharmaceutical agents (Table 1). Although each factor is discussed individually, they usually operate concurrently to provide photoprotection.

While this chapter stresses the use of topical sunscreens, other factors noted in Table 1 are often of equal if not greater import. Accordingly, these will also be briefly discussed.

I. ENDOGENOUS CUTANEOUS COMPONENTS

A. Keratin

The outermost layer of the epidermis consists of the fibrous protein keratin and its amorphous matrix lipids. Keratin, a disulfide-rich protein, absorbs photons in the UVC and UVB ranges. There is great regional variation in the thickness of the keratinous stratum corneum at various body sites such as eyelids and palms. This is reflected in the ease with which eyelids can become swollen following sun exposure, while the palms are virtually never involved.

Major portions of this chapter have been excerpted with permission from Harber, L. and Bickers, D. *Photosensitivity Diseases, Principles of Diagnosis and Treatment*, B. Decker, Publ., Toronto, 1989.

Table 1 Photoprorective Factors Against
Ultraviolet Radiation

Endogenous cutaneous components
 Keratin
 Melanin
 Urocanic acid

Exogenous physical barriers
 Atmospheric ozone
 Pollutants, clouds, fog
 Clothing
 Water

Pharmaceutical agents
 Topically applied
  Photon-absorbing agents
  Photon-blocking agents
 Systemically administered
  Psoralens
  Aminoquinolines
  Beta carotene
  Inhibitors of prostaglandin synthesis
   Acetylsalicylic acid (aspirin)
   Indomethacin

The majority of ultraviolet radiation wavelengths less than 320 nm is absorbed either by the stratum corneum or by the epidermal keratinocyte, which contains potential photon-absorbing chromophores, including RNA, DNA, and urocanic acid. Therefore, relatively few impinging photons of UVB (5–10% in the 290–310 nm range) penetrate the upper epidermis sufficiently to reach the viable basal cell layer and the superficial dermal vasculature.

Conversely, considerable transmission of radiation of wavelengths above 330 nm occurs through the epidermis. Transmission of UVB is reduced by both the scattering and the absorbing properties of keratin in the stratum corneum. A clinical application is noted in patients with vitiligo, who can minimize the intense pain and redness often associated with outdoor activities by gradually increasing their daily sun exposure; this increases the thickness of their stratum corneum (keratin) without associated activity of melanocytes.

B. Melanin

Melanin, a brownish-black, nonhomogeneous pigment, is a heteropolymer synthesized in specialized epidermal cells, the melanocytes. The amount of cutaneous melanin ranges from virtually zero in albino skin to slightly less than one gram in the body of an adult black person. The differences arise primarily from variations in the amounts of melanin synthesized by a relatively fixed number of melanocytes. In other words, the number of melanocytes in a black individual's skin is essentially identical to that found in white skin. Differences in melanosome size are observed in various races, which also influence protection effects of melanin.

The mechanism for increased melanin pigmentation following ultraviolet radiation appears to involve at least two distinct types of reactions: new pigment formation (delayed tanning), and immediate pigment darkening (immediate tanning).

New Pigment Formation

Enhanced activity of tyrosinase followed by new melanin synthesis leads to delayed tanning, which is visible 48 to 72 h after exposure as a "tan." In addition, ultraviolet radiation induces proliferation of melanocytes, resulting in increased numbers of such cells in irradiated skin (1). The melanin formed within the melanocyte is transferred by pinocytosis to the keratinocyte and accumulates above the nuclear membrane. The action spectrum for new melanin synthesis reaction initially was thought to be primarily in the UVB range, but more recent studies have shown that UVA is also effective in evoking delayed tanning (2,3). However, the efficacy of the UVA in producing the delayed tanning reaction is much less than that of UVB (dose of UVA: 20-40 J/cm^2; dose of UVB: 20-100 mJ/cm^2). Paradoxically, photons of UVC radiation from the highly energetic and potentially more damaging cold quartz mercury vapor light sources are much less potent inducers of melanogenesis. Estrogens also may cause melanization by a different and still unclear mechanism. Nonetheless the increase in melanin noted during pregnancy probably results from increased tyrosinase activity.

Immediate Pigment Darkening

The second type of melanization does not require the synthesis of new pigment, but entails oxidation of previously synthesized melanin pigment to produce immediate tanning. Described by Meirowsky (4), this immediate melanization reaction occurs within minutes following exposure to a broad spectrum of solar radiation (UVA, visible light, or infrared radiation). The Meirowsky phenomenon is most readily observed in Caucasians with dark complexions (skin types III and IV). This reaction is the result of photo-oxidation of previously synthesized melanin that produces more light opaque, semiquinone-like free radical material that often appears more grayish than brown (5).

C. Urocanic Acid

Urocanic acid is synthesized in epidermal cells by means of the deamination of the amino acid histidine within keratinocytes. Following ultraviolet exposure, an increase in its synthesis occurs (6,7). Urocanic acid exists in human epidermis as the trans isomer. After absorption of UVB radiation, the trans isomer of urocanic acid is converted to the cis isomer (8). The way in which this photomediated isomerization results in photoprotection is unknown. Studies revealing a similarity of the action spectra for the immunoregulatory effects of ultraviolet radiation and synthesis of urocanic acid as well as studies of the effect of urocanic acid isomers on immune function suggest that this biochemical product of irradiation plays a major role in the overall organism response to sun exposure.

Thus the epidermis is composed of at least two types of cells that provide functional photoprotection: the melanocytes, which manufacture melanin, and the keratinocytes, which synthesize keratin and urocanic acid. Both these biochemical products offer significant protection against ultraviolet radiation.

II. EXOGENOUS PHYSICAL BARRIERS

A. Atmospheric Ozone

Atmospheric ozone (O_3), formed in the stratosphere, absorbs large amounts of UVB radiation (290–320 nm) and still larger amounts of UVC radiation (200–290 nm) (9). It is thus a superb photoprotective agent. However, it absorbs little or no UVA or visible radiation.

Ozone is an unstable, faintly blue gas with a readily detectable acrid odor. The odor can be noted with ease when a hot or cold quartz mercury vapor lamp is ignited in a small room (the 185 nm photons convert oxygen to ozone). Since ozone is a primary irritant to mucous membranes of the nose, lungs, and conjunctivae, adequate ventilation is essential when light sources that emit this gas are used.

Most ozone is found in the stratosphere, 15 to 35 km above sea level, where it may reach a concentration of 10 parts per million (ppm). This amount is exceedingly minute: if it were compressed into a single layer it would form a band less than 3 mm thick. This very fine barrier, however, is critical to life on Earth. Though less striking than its absorption of UVC, it remains superbly effective as an absorber of photons of UVB. This can be demonstrated by the fact that at 300 nm the extraterrestrial flux (concentration) of UVB is twenty times that reaching the Earth's surface (10).

For presently unexplained reasons, a decrease has been noted in the ozone layer (a "black hole") above the South Pole. A 5% reduction in the ozone level at Antarctica has been reported by Australian and American geologists to the alarm of international organizations (11). This black hole presently poses a planetary environmental crisis.

The protective effect of ozone against UVB sunburn erythema can also be correlated with the time of day that sun exposure occurs. At noon, for example, the sun is for practical purposes directly overhead (a zenith angle of 0 degrees). As shown in Figure 1, solar radiation at this time of day passes through less stratospheric ozone (x) than at 4:00 P.M., when the radiation is angulated and so passes through more stratospheric ozone (2x). That ozone is such an effective natural sunscreen during the summer in temperate regions can be shown by demonstrating a fourfold increase in exposure time required at 4:00 P.M. to obtain an erythema exposure similar to that obtained at noon. Thus, the simple measure of maximizing sun exposure in the early morning and late afternoon hours will permit even the most sensitive persons in temperate climates to enjoy sunshine for some period of time daily. In a temperate zone, no sunburn for practical purposes results from exposure of a type III (see Section I.B) individual to sunlight at zenith angles less than 20 degrees and more than 70 degrees, because of the increased amount of ozone that photons must traverse.

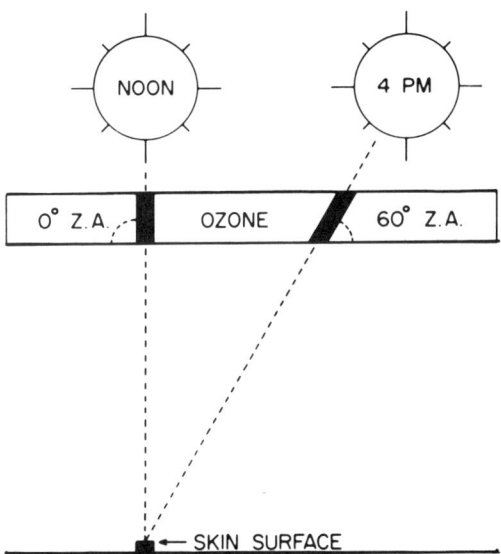

Figure 1 The amount of ozone through which ultraviolet radiation passes increases with the zenith angle (ZA). There is accordingly less hazard from ultraviolet radiation if one avoids sun exposure in the noon time region.

Much concern has recently arisen regarding the use of agents such as the chlorofluorocarbons in aerosol propellant form, which lower the concentration of stratospheric ozone (12,13). It has been demonstrated that cleavage of the chlorofluorocarbons by solar radiation releases free halogens (chlorine, fluorine) that selectively combine with ozone. Theoretical considerations suggest that these halogens, which are still widely used in refrigerants and other nonaerosol products outside the borders of the United States, could contribute to the attenuation of the ozone layer. This would lead to increased penetration of more damaging wavelengths of UVC and UVB radiation. It has been estimated that a 1% decrease in ozone concentration could increase human skin cancer by as much as 2-4%.

B. Pollutants, Clouds, and Fog

Dirt and other particulate matter in the atmosphere reduce the intensity of the ultraviolet and visible light reaching the Earth's surface. In fact, it is estimated that about half of the stratospheric UVB reaches the Earth's surface while the other half is scattered in the atmosphere (14).

Other atmospheric factors, such as the water content of clouds and fog, also scatter ultraviolet radiation but absorb little of it (15). However, clouds and fog strongly absorb infrared radiation and thus diminish the warmth associated with sun exposure. This effect can result in severe sunburn on cloudy days when the ambient temperature may seem cool even though large amounts of ultraviolet radiation are transmitted through the clouds and are absorbed by the skin.

It must be strongly emphasized that snow reflects as much as 85% of the UVB radiation. Accordingly it is not surprising that severe sunburn may occur in midwinter, particularly to those skiing between high mountain ranges.

C. Clothing

Clothing and shelter provide protection against ultraviolet radiation as physical barriers. Staying indoors between 11 A.M. and 3 P.M. (Daylight Savings Time) is helpful in avoiding maximum UVR intensity. Clothing may be only partially effective, depending upon the thickness and weave of the material as well as the color. Dark clothing is an excellent absorber of infrared radiation, often making the individual more uncomfortable by raising body temperature. Therefore, in hot weather, dark garments should be loose fitting to permit the circulation of air and the evaporation of perspiration, which enhance cooling.

D. Water

Pure water permits the transmission of large amounts of ultraviolet radiation and therefore does not provide photoprotection. Because water does absorb in the infrared range, the skin may feel cool and yet be exposed to damaging ultraviolet radiation. While swimming in cool water, a bather may unknowingly be exposed to excessive amounts of UVB. Although not completely protective, "water-resistant" topical sunscreens are advised, particularly when swimming in pools.

III. PHARMACEUTICAL AGENTS

Erythema following sun exposure is due to both ultraviolet B radiation (UVB) and ultraviolet A radiation (UVA). Early erythema studies by Hausser more than sixty years ago and those more recently done confirm that approximately 1000-fold more UVA than UVB energy is required to elicit erythema in human skin (16-20). However, because the total UVA energy reaching the Earth exceeds the UVB by 10- to 100-fold, UVA radiation may constitute 10% or more of the total ultraviolet radiation reaching the skin; during the hours around dawn and dusk, for example, UVA may account for as much as 90% of the ultraviolet radiation reaching the skin. Accordingly, protection against both UVB and UVA should be considered when evaluating a topical sunscreen preparation.

In recent years a new means of predicting the effectiveness of topical sunscreens has been established. The sun protection factor (SPF) of a sunscreen is an experimentally derived number intended to provide the consumer with information concerning sunscreen products, giving an approximation of its protective effect on the skin against UVB radiation. No similar convention has been agreed upon for UVA.

The SPF value is defined as the ratio of the dose of energy required to produce minimal erythema or sunburn (MED) through a sunscreen product film, as compared with the amount of energy to produce the same MED without any treatment (21). The following equation describes this ratio:

$$SPF = \frac{MED \text{ of protected skin}}{MED \text{ of unprotected skin}}$$

A. Topically Applied Agents

Topically applied chemicals that act as sun protectors (Table 2) are widely utilized and currently offer the most convenient means of protecting human skin against sunburn and other chronic pathologic effects of ultraviolet radiation (22-24). When applied to the skin, sunscreens remain primarily in the stratum corneum. Their effectiveness is based upon two different mechanisms of action: the absorption of photons (Group 1) and the reflecting and scattering of photons (Group 2).

Table 2   Topically Applied Sunscreens

Photon-absorbing agents
    Para-amino benzoic acid (PABA)
    PABA esters
    Salicylates
    Cinnamates
    Benzophenones
    Dibenzoylmethanes

Photon-blocking agents
    Zinc oxide
    Titanium dioxide
    Calamine
    Neocalamine

B.   Photon-Absorbing Agents

UVB Absorbers

The most extensively used light-absorbing sunscreen preparations contain para-amino benzoic acid (PABA) and its derivatives (25–27). PABA esters such as octyldimethyl (Padimate O, Escalol 507), glyceryl (Escalol 106), and amyldimethyl (Padimate A, Escalol 506) are widely used. PABA and its derivatives are readily available, inexpensive, and relatively free of side effects; however, allergic contact sensitization, photoallergic contact dermatitis, staining of clothing, and a stinging sensation may occur in the skin shortly after application. Contaminants in their synthesis such as benzocaine also have been reported to cause adverse responses. The absorption spectrum for PABA and several of its esters closely approximates the UVB action spectrum for erythema. Thus, the chemical absorption of UVB by PABA and PABA esters in the stratum corneum prevents transmission of these rays to the deeper layers of the skin and prevents sunburn.

The protective effect of sunscreens is dependent upon more than the absorption spectrum of the compound. A second determinant of effectiveness is substantivity, or the sunscreen's resistance to removal from the skin by perspiration, swimming, and washing. For labeling purposes, substantivity can be judged by a modification of SPF testing methods. A *water-resistant* SPF is determined after two 20-minute immersions in water, while a *waterproof* SPF is determined after four such immersions (80 minutes total).

Other chemical groups used as sunscreens are the salicylates, the cinnamates, and the benzophenones (28). The cinnamates and salicylates absorb in the UVB and the UVA, and are somewhat effective.

UVA Absorbers

Photoprotection in the UVA spectrum has only recently become of interest in clinical and basic science. UVA radiation currently is under study because of its possible relationship to neoplasia, aging, and immunologic changes in the skin.

Concern for these risks has led several investigators to evaluate the need for protection against UVA. Early studies by Parrish, Willis, and others indicate that approximately 1,000 times as many photons of UVA are required to produce erythema compared with UVB (29–31). However, because UVA penetrates the Earth's atmosphere more readily than UVB or UVC, the Earth's surface receives an average of 10 to 100 times more UVA than UVB (depending upon the season of the year). Therefore, the contribution of UVA to erythema and to possible solar damage can be considerable, in spite of the fact that it is much less damaging per unit photon.

In the early morning and late afternoon, when much of UVB radiation is being absorbed by atmospheric ozone, solar erythema is due to a disproportionately large percentage of UVA. The relative contributions of UVB and UVA to erythema as determined by the angle of the sun are shown in Table 3.

In an effort to develop sunscreens that protect against UVA, chemicals with broad (UVA and UVB) absorption spectra have been added to sunscreen products (Table 4). The two most commonly used ingredients for this purpose are the benzophenones and the dibenzoylmethanes. Nc technique analogous to SPF testing is presently accepted as standard for evaluating UVA photoprotection (32). It is likely that as interest in this area grows, standardization and regulatory requirements for labelling will be codified.

Table 3 Relative Erythemogenesis of Solar UVB and UVA as a Function of Solar Zenith Angle

	Zenith angle			
	0° (noon)	30°	50°	70°
Approximate total UVA irradiance at 320–400 nm (in mW/cm^2)	5.1	3.6	1.8	0.3
Time (h) for MED from solar UVA alone (30 J/cm^2)	1.6	2.3	4.6	–
Time for MED from solar UVB alone	16.0 min	34.0 min	3.0	–
Percent of 1 MED due to solar UVA	14%	25%	39%	–

Table 4   Selected Sunscreening Chemicals that Absorb UVA Radiation

Agent	Concentration (%)
4-Isopropyl-dibenzoylmethane (Eusolex 8020)	5
Methylbenzylidene camphor	5
2-Phenylbenzimidazole-5-sulfonic acid	2
Phenylpyridylpropaneione	5
2-Ethyl-hexyl-*p*-methoxycinnamate	5
2-Hydroxy-4-methoxy-benzophenone (oxybenzone)	3–7
4-Tert. butyl-4-methoxydibenzoylmethane (Parsol 1789)	2–3
2-Hydroxy-4-methoxy-benzophenone-5-sulfonic acid	3–5
2-Ethyl-hexyl-4-phenylbenzophenone-5-sulfonic acid	3–5

Photon-Blocking Agents

A different but often effective approach to sunprotection is the use of sun-screens of Group 2. These are opaque materials that reflect or scatter ultraviolet and visible radiation. Titanium dioxide (TiO_2) is the most widely used, but talc ($MgSiO_2$), calamine (FeO_2), bentonite, kaolin, and zinc oxide (ZnO) share its properties. Unfortunately, these agents, although effective, are often unaccept-able to many photosensitive patients, since they are not transparent, have a "gritty" consistency, and may leave a masklike residue on the skin.

C. Systemically Administered Agents

Psoralens

8-Methoxypsoralen and trimethylpsoralen afford photoprotection primarily by stimulating increased melanin formation and, to a lesser extent, by an increased keratin synthesis and thickening of the stratum corneum. Hypermelanosis fol-lows the phototoxic reaction associated with their use in combination with UVA. Patients are advised to ingest the drug 1.5 to 2 hours before going out-doors. An initial 15-minute exposure is recommended, with increased increments of daily exposure until 30–45 minutes of sunlight is tolerated. Extreme caution is required, since severe vesicular and bullous reactions may follow excessive sun exposure.

    We believe that under all but the most unusual circumstances psoralens do not provide an appropriate means for the average nonphotosensitive individual to obtain a cosmetically acceptable photoprotective tan. Indeed the damage resulting from the phototoxic reaction to the psoralen-UVA (PUVA) combination has been demonstrated to increase the risk of cutaneous malignancy in patients treated with PUVA for psoriasis (33).

Psoralens are not advised for routine use in patients desiring a quick "cosmetic tan," but may be cautiously used in numerous photodermatoses (34–36).

Aminoquinolines

The antimalarial drugs, including chloroquine (Aralen), hydroxychloroquine (Plaquenil), and quinacrine (Atabrine), are effective in increasing tolerance to sunlight in patients with abnormal photosensitivities (e.g., patients with lupus erythematosus and polymorphous light eruption). The mechanisms of action of these drugs are unknown; however, they do not decrease the erythema response of normal individuals.

The major limiting factor in the use of the antimalarial drugs is their toxicity. Cutaneous side effects include lichenoid drug eruptions, exfoliative erythroderma, and exacerbation of psoriasis and porphyria cutanea tarda, to name several. However, the toxic effects of major concern are those related to the eye. The antimalarials cause changes in both the cornea and the retina. Corneal deposits of the drugs are usually asymptomatic, and they soon resolve upon discontinuation of the medication. Retinopathy is the primary limiting factor in the use of these drugs. Because of the irreversibility of these toxic effects, the early detection of retinopathy is essential. It has recently been established that field-testing the paracentral area may provide early confirmation of developing retinopathy.

Beta Carotene

The excessive ingestion of carotene, as naturally found in tomatoes or in nutrient supplements, leads to a yellowing appearance of the skin. This approach to adding pigmentation to the skin is relatively harmless but has been disappointing in that there appears to be very little if any increase in photoprotection.

Inhibitors of Prostaglandin Synthesis

Acetylsalicylic Acid (Aspirin) Although it has excellent analgesic properties and may influence early (sunburn) erythema because of its inhibitory effects on prostaglandin synthesis, acetylsalicylic acid has demonstrated no significant photoprotective effect against erythema evaluated 24 hours after exposure (37).

Indomethacin The photoprotective effects of indomethacin in delaying the onset and reducing the intensity of UVB erythema appear similar to those of aspirin (38). There is no evidence that they protect against damage to DNA, even when release of prostaglandins and subsequent erythema is inhibited (39).

Table 5, disseminated by the FDA in 1978, lists sunscreening and sunblocking agents considered to be safe and effective for both UVB and UVA. Commercial names of broad groups are noted in Table 6. Brand names of selected agents are listed according to their photon-absorbing and photon-blocking properties (Tables 4, 7, and 8). The structural formulas of selected sunscreen drug families are shown in Figure 2.

Table 5   Topical Sunscreening and Sunblocking Agents Considered to be Safe and Effective (Category 1)

Amino benzoic acid

Cinoxate

Diethanolamine *p*-methoxycinnamate

Digalloyl trioleate

Dioxybenzone

Ethyl 4-aminobenzoate

Ethyl 4-[*bis*(hydroxypropyl)] aminobenzoate

2-Ethyl-hexyl 2-cyano-3,3-dephenylacrylate

Ethyl-hexyl *p*-methoxycinnamate

2-Ethyl-hexyl salicylate

Glycerol aminobenzoate

Homosalate

Lawsone with dihydroxyacetone

Menthyl anthranilate

Oxybenzone

Padimate A

Padimate O

2-Phenylbenzimidazole-5-sulfonic acid

Red petrolatum

Sulisobenzone

Titanium dioxide

Triethanolamine salicylate

Source: From Ref. 23, pp. 38210–38230.

Table 6 Selected Properties of Some Brand-Name Sunscreens Under Outdoor Conditions

Trade name	Ingredients	Type of sunscreen	(SPF) Outdoor sunlight	Substantivity (resistance to sweating)[a]
PABA sunscreens:				
PreSun-15	5% PABA in 50%–70%	Clear lotion	10–12	Excellent
PABA ester sunscreens:				
Block out	3.3% Isoamyl-p-N,N-dimethyl aminobenzoate (padimate-A)	Lotion/gel	6	Good
Pabafilm	3.3% Isoamyl-p-N,N-dimethyl aminobenzoate (padimate-A)	Lotion/gel	4–6	Good
Sundown	3.3% Isoamyl-p-N,N dimethyl aminobenzoate (padimate-A)	Lotion	4–6	Good
Original Eclipse	3.5% Padimate-A + 3.0% octyldimethyl PABA	Lotion	4–6	Fair
Sea & Ski	3.3% Octyldimethyl PABA	Cream	4	Fair
PABA-ester combinations sunscreens:				
Coppertone Supershade-15	7% Octyldimethyl PABA + 3% oxybenzone	Milky lotion	10–12	Excellent
Total Eclipse	2.5% Glyceryl PABA + 2.5% octyldimethyl PABA + 2.5% oxybenzone	Milky lotion	10–14	Excellent
PreSun-15 (water-resistant)	8% Padimate-O + 3% oxybenzone	Milky lotion	10–14	Excellent
Clinique-19	Phenyl-benzimidazole-5-sulfonic acid + 2.5% octyldimethyl PABA	Milky lotion	14	Good
Sundown-15[b] block	7% Padimate-O + octyl-alicylate + 4% oxybenzone	Milky lotion	10–11	Excellent
Bain de Soleil	7.0% Padimate-O + 2.5% oxybenzone + 5.0% dioxybenzone	White cream	9	Excellent

Table 6 (Continued)

Trade name	Ingredients	Type of sunscreen	(SPF) Outdoor sunlight	Substantivity (resistance to sweating)[a]
Elizabeth Arden Suncare Creme-15	Padimate-O + oxybenzone	White cream	14	Good
Estee Lauder-15	Phenyl-benzimidazole-5-sulfonic acid + di-methyl PABA	White cream	9	Good
Shiseido-15	6.5% Titanium dioxide + 2.5% octyldimethyl PABA + 0.3% benzophenone-3	Lotion	8–10	Good
Non-PABA sunscreens:				
Piz Buin-8[c]	5% Ethyl-hexyl-p-metho-oxycinnamate + 1.5% 4 tert. Butyl-4-methoxybenzoyl methane	Cream	10–12	Excellent
TIScreen-15	3% 2-Hydroxy-4-metho-benzophenone	Milky lotion	10–12	Excellent
UVAL	10% 2-Hydroxy-4-methoxybenzophenone-5-sulfonic	Milky lotion	4	Poor
Coppertone	8% Homomenthylsalicylate	Lotion	2	Poor
Piz Buin-12	4.5% Octyl-methoxycinnamate + 4.5% zinc oxide + 4.5% talc + 2.2% benzophenone-3	Milky lotion	12–14	Excellent
Sunblock sunscreens:				
A-Fil		Cream	4–6	Good
RV Paque	Titanium dioxide + zinc oxide + talc, kaolin,	Cream	6–8	Good
Covermark	iron oxide, or red veterinary petrolatum	Cream	4–6	Good
Clinique		Cream	4–6	Good

[a]SPF value retained: Excellent = over 90–100%; Good = 75–90%; Fair = 50–70%; Poor = less than 50%.
[b]Ingredients may include octyldimethyl PABA + oxybenzone.
Source: Modified from Pathak et al.
[c]Not currently available in the United States.
Source: M. Pathak, personal communication, 1988.

Table 7 Selected Sunscreens Containing Photon Absorbers

PABA, PABA esters	Combination benzophenone and PABA esters	Non-PABA benzophenones and cinnamates
PreSun	Supershade–15	Piz Buin 8, 12, and 15
PABANOL	Sundown–15	TI-Screen
Blockout	3M–15	UVAL
PABA Film	Clinique–19	Solbar
Sundown–8	PreSun–15	Marbert Sun Cream–8
Sea & Ski	Elizabeth Arden–15	
Sunbrella	Bain de Soleil	

Source: From M. Pathak, personal communication, 1988.

Table 8 Selected Sunscreens Containing Photon Blocking Agents (Recommended for Photosensitive Patients)

Trade name	Ingredients (all)	Type of sunscreen
Physical Sunscreens:		
A-Fil		Cream
RV Paque		Cream
Shadow	Titanium dioxide + zinc oxide + talc, kaolin, iron oxide, or red veterinary petrolatum	Cream
Reflecta		Cream
Covermark		Cream
Clinique		Cream
Solar cream		Cream

Source: Modified from M. Pathak, personal communication, 1988.

Family	Members
p-Aminobenzoates	Dimethyl
	Ethyl
	Isobutyl
	Monoglyceryl
o-Aminobenzoates or anthranilates	Benzyl
	Cyclohexanyl
	Lauryl
	Menthyl
	Phenyl
	Triethanolamine
Salicylates (o-hydroxybenzoic acid)	Amyl
	Benzyl
	Bornyl
	1.3-Butyleneglycol mono
	Glyceryimononohomomenthyl
	Isoamyl
	Menthyl
	Parathymol
	Phenyl (salol)
	Triethanolamine
	Thymol
	Salicylic acid ester of a polyalcohol
Pyrrones	Benzyl cinnamate
	β-Umbelliferone acetic acid
	3-Methyl umbelliferone
	1.3-Butylene-glycol cinnamate
	3-Methyl umbelliferone acetic acid
	Cinnamic acid
	Coumaric (o-hydroxycinnamic) acid
	Daphnetin or dihydroxycoumarin
	Daphnetic-8-ethyl ether
	Esculin (aesculin)
	Esculetin or 6,7-dihydroxycoumarin
	Ethyl umbelliferone
	Homomenthyl cinnamate
	2-Hydroxy-3-methoxycinnamic acid
	3-Methoxy-o-coumaric acid
	Methyl umbelliferone acetate
	Methyl esculetin
	3-Phenylcoumarin
	Phenyl cinnamic nitrite
	Umbelliferone (7-hydroxycoumarin)
	Also. esculin-quinine condensation products
Naphtholsulfonic acid	Naphthol sulfonate
	1,5-Naphtholsulfonic acid
	2,6-Naphtholsulfonic acid
	2,8-Naphtholsulfonic acid
	3.2-Naphtholsulfonic acid
Napthoic acid	β-Oxynaphthoic acid
	α,β-Oxynaphthoic acid
	2-Hydroxy-2-naphthoic acid

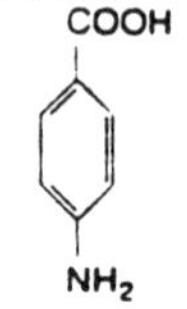

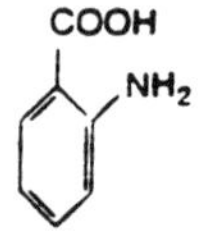

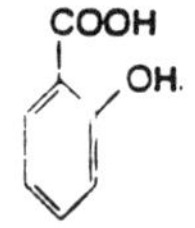

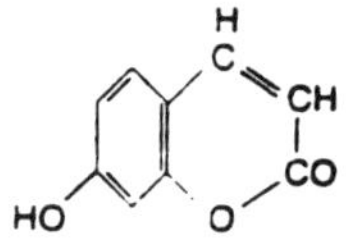

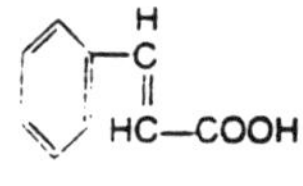

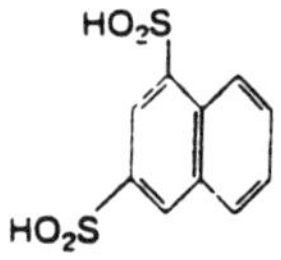

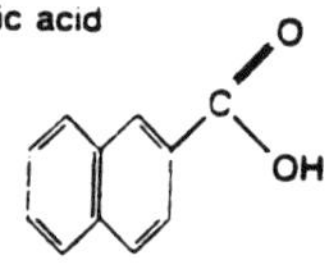

Figure 2   Structural formulas of selected sunscreens. (From Ref. 24.)

IV. PEDIATRIC RECOMMENDATIONS

Studies concerning photoprotection indicate that the risk of developing skin cancer is increased by excessive sun exposure during childhood (40-44). As a large proportion of the damage from solar radiation that has been linked to cutaneous melanoma is incurred during the first 10 to 20 years of life, sun protection for children is particularly important (45).

Recommendations for children are substantially the same as have been mentioned throughout this chapter, such as wearing protective clothing, being careful about reflective surfaces including snow, sand, and water, as well as avoiding tanning salons. In addition, use of sunscreens with a minimum SPF of 15 is advised (46). Protecting children from excessive sun exposure is important not only to prevent the deleterious effects of ultraviolet radiation during critical years, but also to teach them habits of sun protection that will continue to minimize skin damage in later life (47).

REFERENCES

1. Rosdahl, I. K. and Szabo, G. Mitotic activity of epidermal melanocytes in UV-irradiated mouse skin. *J. Invest. Dermatol.*, *70*:143-148 (1978).
2. Willis, I., Kligman, A., and Epstein, J. Effects of long ultraviolet rays on human skin: photoprotective or photoaugmentative. *J. Invest. Dermatol.*, *59*:416-420 (1972).
3. Jimbow, K., Kaidbey, L. H., Pathak, M. A., et al. Melanin pigmentation stimulated by UV-B, UV-A and psoralen. *J. Invest. Dermatol.*, *62*:548 (1974).
4. Meirowsky, E. A critical review of pigment research in the last hundred years. *Br. J. Dermatol.*, *52*:205-217 (1940).
5. Pathak, M. A. and Stratton, K. A study of the free radicals in human skin before and after exposure to light. *Arch. Biochem. Biophys.*, *123*:468-476 (1968).
6. Baden, H. P. and Pathak, M. A. Trans to cis isomerization of urocanic acid in the skin. *J. Invest. Dermatol.*, *48*:11-17 (1967).
7. Anglin, J. G. and Batten, W. H. Studies on cis-urocanic acid. *J. Invest. Dermatol.*, *50*:463-466 (1968).
8. Baden, H. P., Pathak, M. A., and Butler, D. Trans to cis isomerization of urocanic acid. *Nature*, *210*:732-733 (1966).
9. Dauvillier, A. The photochemical origin of life, *Scripta Technica* (trans). Academic Press, New York (1965), p. 96.
10. Campbell I. M. *Energy and the Atmosphere*, 2nd ed., John Wiley, Chichester (1986), p. 13.
11. Longstreth, J. D. Ultraviolet radiation and melanoma with a special focus on assessing the stratospheric ozone depletion. EPA Publication 1987: 400/1-87/001 D.

12. Maugh, T. G., 2nd. The threat to ozone is real, increasing. *Science, 206*: 1167–1168 (1979).
13. Maugh, T. G., 2nd. Ozone depletion would have dire effect. *Science, 207*: 394–395 (1980).
14. Daniels, F. Jr. Physical factors in sun exposure. *Arch. Dermatol., 85*:358–361 (1962).
15. Smith, R. C. and Tyler, J. E. Transmission of solar radiation into natural waters, *Photochemical and Photobiological Reviews* (K. C. Smith, ed.), Plenum, New York (1976), pp. 117–155.
16. Hausser, K. W. and Vahle, W. Sunburn and suntanning, *The Biologic Effects of Ultraviolet Radiation* (F. Urbach, ed.), Pergamon Press, Oxford (1969), p. 3.
17. Parrish, J. A., et al. *Biological Effects of Ultraviolet Radiation with Emphasis on Human Responses to Longwave Ultraviolet*, UVA. Plenum Press, New York (1978), p. 107.
18. Parrish, J. A., et al. Cutaneous effects of pulsed nitrogen gas laser irradiation. *J. Invest. Dermatol., 67*:603–608 (1976).
19. Whitman, G. B., et al. Comparative study of erythema response to UVA radiation in guinea pigs and humans. *Photochem. Photobiol., 42*:399–403 (1985).
20. Pathak, M. A. Sunscreens: Topical and systemic approaches for the prevention of acute and chronic sun-induced skin reactions. *Dermatol. Clin., 4*:321–334 (1986).
21. Pathak, M. A., et al. Sunlight and melanin pigmentation, *Photochemical and Photobiological Reviews* (K. C. Smith, ed.), Plenum, New York (1976), pp. 211–213.
22. Abramowitz, M. Sunscreens. *Med. Letter, 30*:61–63 (1988).
23. Gardner, S. Sunscreen drug products for over-the-counter human use. *Fed. Reg., 43*:38206–38269 (1978).
24. Giese, A. C., Christensen, E., and Jeppon, J. Absorption spectra of some sunscreens for skin preparations. *J. Am. Pharm. Assoc., 39*:30–36 (1950).
25. Pathak, M. A., Fitzpatrick, T. B., and Frenk, E. Evaluation of topical agents that prevent sunburn: superiority of para-aminobenzoic acid and its esters in ethyl alcohol. *N. Engl. J. Med., 280*:1459–1463 (1969).
26. Willis, I. and Kligman, A. M. Aminobenzoic acid and its esters. *Arch. Dermatol., 102*:405–417 (1970).
27. Pathak, M. A. Sunscreens and their use in the preventative treatment of sunlight-induced skin damage. *J. Dermatol. Surg. Oncol., 13*:739–750 (1987).
28. Knox, J. M., Guin, J., and Cockerell, E. G. Benzophenones: ultraviolet light absorbing agents. *J. Invest. Dermatol., 29*:435–444 (1957).
29. Willis, I. and Cylus, L. UVA erythema in skin: Is it a sunburn? *J. Invest. Dermatol., 68*:128–129 (1977).
30. Hawk, J. L. M., Black, A. K., Jaeneck, K. F., et al. Increased concentrations

of arachidonic acid, prostaglandins E_2, D_2, and 60oxo-F-F_1 and histamine in skin following ultraviolet-A irradiation. *J. Invest. Dermatol., 80*:494–499 (1983).

31. Regan, J. D. and Parrish, J. A. (eds.). *The Science of Photomedicine*. Plenum, New York (1982).
32. Chew, S., DeLeo, V. A., and Harber, L. C. An animal model for evaluation of topical photoprotection against ultraviolet-A (320–380 nm). *J. Invest. Dermatol., 89*:410–414 (1987).
33. Stern, R. S., Scotto, J., and Fears, T. R. Psoriasis and susceptibility to non-melanoma skin cancer. *J. Am. Acad. Dermatol., 12*:67–73 (1985).
34. Pfau, R. G., Hood, A. F., and Morison, W. L. Photoageing: the role of UVB, solar-simulated UVB, visible and psoralen UVA radiation. *Br. J. Dermatol., 114*:319–327 (1986).
35. Morison, W. L. In vivo effects of psoralens plus longwave ultraviolet radiation on immunity. *Natl. Cancer. Inst. Monogr., 66*:243–246 (1984).
36. Morison, W. L. and Strickland, P. T. Environmental UVA radiation and eye protection during PUVA therapy. *J. Am. Acad. Dermatol., 9*:522–525 (1983).
37. Dinarello, C. A. Interleukin-1 and the effects of cyclooxygenase inhibitors on its biological activities. *Bull. NY Acad. Med., 65*:80–92 (1989).
38. Krane, S. M., Dayer, J. M., Simon, L. S., and Byrne, S. Mononuclear cell-conditioned medium containing mononuclear cell factor (MCF), homologous with interleukin-1, stimulates collagen and fibronectin synthesis by adherent rheumatoid synovial cells: effects of prostaglandin E_2 and indomethacin. *Collagen Rel. Res., 5*:99–117 (1985).
39. Konturek, S. J., Kwiecien, N., Obtulowicz, W., et al. Effect of carprofen and indomethacin on gastric function, mucosal integrity and generation of prostaglandins in men. *Hepato-Gastroenterol., 29*:267–280 (1982).
40. Lew, R. A., Sober, A. J., Cook, N., et al. Sunburn, sun exposure, and melanoma skin cancer. *J. Dermatol. Surg. Oncol., 9*:981–986 (1983).
41. Rhodes, A. R., Weinstock, M. A., Fitzpatrick, T. B., et al. Risk factors for cutaneous melanoma: A practical method of recognizing predisposed individuals. *JAMA, 258*:3146–3154 (1987).
42. Green, A. Sun exposure and the risk of melanoma. *Aust. J. Dermatol., 25*:99–102 (1984).
43. Fitzpatrick, T. B. Abstracts: Sun protection for life in the high risk population. *J. Dermatol. Surg. Oncol., 11*:785 (1985).
44. Holman, C. D. J., Armstrong, B. K., and Heenan, P. J. Relationship of cutaneous malignant melanoma to individual sunlight-exposure habits. *JNCI, 76*:403–414 (1986).
45. Hurwitz, S. The sun and sunscreen protection: Recommendations for children. *J. Dermatol. Surg. Oncol., 14*:657–660 (1988).
46. Stern, R. S., Weinstein, M. C., and Baker, S. G. Risk reduction for non-melanoma skin cancer with childhood sunscreen use. *Arch. Dermatol., 122*:537–545 (1986).

47. Goldsmith, M. F. Medical news and perspectives: Paler is better, say skin cancer fighters. *JAMA, 257*:893–894 (1987).

48. Noonan, F. P., DeFabo, E. C., and Morrison, H. Cis-urocanic acid, a product formed by ultraviolet radiation of the skin, initiates an antigen-presenting defect in splenic dendritic cells in vivo. *J. Invest. Dermatol., 90*: 92–99.

11
Sun Protection Factors: Comparative Techniques and Selection of Ultraviolet Sources

NICHOLAS J. LOWE *Skin Research Foundation of California, Santa Monica, California, and UCLA School of Medicine, Los Angeles, California*

I. SUNSCREEN GUIDELINES IN THE UNITED STATES

The *Federal Register* published in 1978 (1) established guidelines for the formulation and evaluation of sunscreens marketed in the United States. These guidelines were re-evaluated in 1988 and a further revised monograph is anticipated in the near future from the Food and Drug Administration (FDA).

The 1978 publication suggested sun protection factors (SPF) be categorized according to the level of protection afforded, ranging from minimal sun protection with an SPF of 2-4 up to an ultra-sun protection maximum SPF of 15.

These guidelines suggested that no product exceeded a maximum SPF level of 15. However, recently many products have been claimed to have SPF numbers much higher than 15, some as high as 50. These higher SPF numbers have been achieved mainly by increasing the concentration of sunscreening chemical to the maximum allowed under the monograph guidelines. Other products have improved their substantivity and SPF numbers by modification of vehicle.

Some of the studies discussed in this chapter were supported by a grant from the Skin Research Foundation of California, Los Angeles, California.

II. SUN PROTECTION FACTOR (SPF) DETERMINATION IN THE UNITED STATES

The *Federal Register* gives the precise instructions on performance of SPF evaluation. The sun protection factor is defined as:

$$SPF = \frac{\text{Minimal Erythema Dose in sunscreen-protected skin}}{\text{Minimal Erythema Dose in non-sunscreen-protected skin}}$$

Selection of subjects is of great importance for the determination of SPF. In general, skin types 1 to 3 are the ideal skin type to utilize for these investigations (see Table 1).

Darker skin types require much longer irradiance times. In general, the longer the irradiance, the more likelihood of more variable minimal erythema dose (MED) determinations.

In my laboratory, I prefer to utilize the lower back previously non-sun-exposed skin for static SPF investigations (1,2). A minimal erythema dose (MED) is first determined. This is the minimum dose of ultraviolet light expressed as joules per cm^2 (J/cm^2) required to produce a minimal uniform skin erythema with clear margins. Light proof adhesive metal foil is used to produce a template that contains 1 cm^2 areas. This is placed on the lower back skin and areas of skin are uncovered at precisely determined times. In this way an accurate MED is determined for each subject on the first day of the study.

The response to the ultraviolet radiation is determined usually 24 hours following the irradiation. From previous experience, we know the approximate MED of each skin type with the solar simulator. The amounts of ultraviolet radiation are then delivered to approximate that anticipated MED time. Increments of 25% ultraviolet time around the anticipated MED are used.

The following day, the sunscreens to be tested are delivered by applying amounts of 2 $\mu g/cm^2$ or 2 $\mu l/cm^2$. These are measured carefully with a measur-

Table 1 Skin Types Determined by Historical Response to Sun

I.	Always burns easily; never tans (sensitive)
II.	Always burns easily; tans minimally (sensitive)
III.	Burns moderately; tans gradually (light brown)
IV.	Burns minimally; always tans well (moderate brown) (normal)
V.	Rarely burns; tans profusely (dark brown) (insensitive)
VI.	Never burns; deeply pigmented (insensitive)

Based on 30–40 minutes sun exposure in early summer without previous sun exposure that season.

ing pipette. The areas will have been previously marked using the template noted above. Since most sunscreen products have a specific gravity of almost unity, the volume measurement of $2 \, \mu l/cm^2$ is usually utilized (1). It is most important that the sunscreen application be very uniform and the technician carefully trained in this technique. Large variations are obtained with irregularly applied amounts of sunscreen.

There have been recent studies to suggest that the average individual applies less than $2 \, \mu l/cm^2$ of sunscreen in regular use (3,4) (see chapter by Gottlieb, Bourget and Lowe for further detailed discussion of this subject). It may be more relevant to apply smaller amounts of sunscreen for SPF determinations as smaller amounts are almost certainly utilized in routine usage by people.

The sunscreens are allowed to dry on the skin for 15 minutes prior to radiation. Again, this does not reflect practical human usage with many individuals. Some sunscreens are highly protective as soon as they are applied. Further investigations are required to determine how rapidly and for how long sunscreens retain their SPF numbers.

After the sunscreens are applied, the volunteer is again irradiated at the sunscreen protected sites with 25% incremental amounts of irradiance based on a preliminary estimation of the SPF number for that sunscreen. By this I mean, we either obtain a spectrophotometric absorption estimate of the expected SPF or, we determine the SPF with carefully measured incremental amounts of irradiance in a small number of volunteer patients. By this means of estimation, excessive ultraviolet burning of a volunteer's skin is avoided.

The volunteers are again examined 24 hours after irradiation. The minimal erythema doses are then determined for both sunscreen-protected, as well as nonprotected skin and the SPF is determined from the ratio of these results.

III. EUROPEAN TESTING

There are several key differences in the details required for SPF determinations between the United States (1) and Europe (5). One clear difference relates to the types of ultraviolet apparatus that are allowed. This is discussed in further detail later in this chapter.

1. Key differences exist between the amounts of application that are allowed. The U.S. monograph recommends $2 \, \mu l/cm^2$ (1). The German DIN recommends $1.5 \, \mu l/cm^2$ (5). This $1.5 \, \mu l$ amount is, incidentally, much closer to the average amount of sunscreen application that we determined most volunteers should use (see Chap. 28).

2. Some other differences between the German DIN and the U.S. FDA guidelines are the different amounts of incremental UV irradiances. The U.S. guidelines suggest that the irradiances are increased by 25% incre-

ments. In the German DIN studies, there is a logarythmic increase as follows: If the initial irradiation time equals 2 minutes, then other irradiance times will be 2.8, 4, 5.6, 8, 11.2, 16, and 22 minutes.

3. In Germany sunscreens are applied 20 minutes prior to irradiation rather than the 15 minutes required in the United States. Sunscreen types and concentration ranges allowed by the U.S. monograph (Table 2) are more restricted than those products allowed in Europe (Table 3).

Table 2 Sunscreens Allowed in United States Under FDA-OTC Panel With Concentration Range

	Approved %
Chemical	
UVA absorbers	
Oxybensone	2–6
Sulisobenzone	5–10
Dioxybenzone	3
Menthyl antranilate	3.5–5
UVB absorbers	
Aminobenzoic acid	5–15
Amyl dimethyl PABA	1–5
2-Ethoxyethyl *p*-methoxycinnamate	1–3
Diethanolamine *p*-methoxycinnamate	8–10
Digalloyl trioleate	2–5
Ethyl 4-bis (hydroxypropyl) aminobenzoate	1–5
2-Ethylhexyl-2-cyano-3,3-diphenyl-acrylate	7–10
Ethylhexyl *p*-methoxycinnamate	2–7.5
2-Ethylhexyl salicylate	3–5
Glyceryl aminobenzoate	2–3
Homomenthyl salicylate	4–25
Lawsone with dihydroxyacetone	0.25 with 3
Octyl dimethyl PABA	1.4–8
2-Penylbenzimidazole-5-sulfonic acid	1.4
Triethanolamine salicylate	5–12
Physical	
Red petrolatum	30–100
Titanium dioxide	2–25

Table 3 Sunscreen Chemicals Used in Europe

European Economic Community chemical name	Maximum % concentration
4-Aminobenzoic acid	5
N,N,N,-trimethyl-4-(2-oxoborn-3-ylidene methyl anilinium methyl sulphate	6
Homosalate	10
Oxybenzone	10
3-Imidazol-4-ylacrylic acid and ethyl ester	2
2-Phenylbenzimidazole-5-sulfonic acid and salts	8
Ethyl-4-bis (hydroxypropyl) aminobenzoate	5
Ethoxylated 4-aminobenzoic acid	10
Amyl 4-dimethylaminobenzoate	5
Glyceryl 1-(4-aminobenzoate)	5
2-Ethylhexyl 4-dimethylaminobenzoate	8
2-Ethylhexyl salicylate	5
3,3,5-Trimethylcyclohexyl-2-acetamido benzoate	2
Potassium cinnamate	2
4-Methoxycinnamic acid salts	8
Propyl 4-methoxycinnamate	3
Salicylic acid salts	2
Amyl 4-methoxycinnamate	10
2-Ethylhexyl 4-methoxycinnamate	10
Cinoxate	5
Digalloyl trioleate	4
Mexenone	4
Sulisobenzone	5
2-Ethylhexyl 2-(4-phenylbenzoyl)-benzoate	10
5-Methyl-2-phenylbenzoxazone	4
Sodium 3,4-dimethoxphenylglyoxylate	5
1,3-bis (4Methoxyphenyl)propane-1,3-dione	6
5-(3,3-Dimethyl-2-norbonylidene)-3-penten-2-one	3
a'-(2-Oxoborn-3-ylidene)-*p*-xylene-2-sulfonic acid	6
a'-(2-Oxoborn-3-ylidene) toluene-4-sulfonic acid and its salts	6
3-(4-Methylbenzylidene)bornan-2-one	6
3-Benzylidenebornana-2-one	6
a-Cyano-4-methoxyclinnamic acid and its hexyl ester	5
1-*p*-Cumenyl-3-phenylpropane-1,3-dione	5
4-Isopropylbenzyl salicylate	4
Cyclohexyl 4-methoxycinnamate	1
1-(40tert-Butylphenyl-3-(4-methoxy-phenyl) propane-1,3-dione	5

IV. TYPES OF ULTRAVIOLET APPARATUS AVAILABLE
FOR SUNSCREEN TESTING

A variety of ultraviolet sources have been used worldwide for sunscreen evaluation. In the United States, the FDA monograph (1) recommends the use of appropriately filtered xenon arc solar simulators for the routine evaluation of sunscreens. However, this monograph does allow the use of alternative ultraviolet sources providing correlation with a variety of sunscreens has been confirmed in comparison studies with an appropriately filtered xenon arc simulator. The West German guidelines (5) (Deutsches Institute fur Nurmung) DIN system recommends the use of an intermediate pressure mercury vapor lamp (Osram Vitalux). This unit does not produce a close solar simulating spectrum as does the xenon arc solar simulator.

A. Xenon Arc Solar Simulators

These sources are available with different lamp outputs. The xenon arc lamp power generally ranges between 150 and 5,000 W. With the 5,000-W sources, water cooling is usually required to reduce damage to reflecting mirrors within the lamp housing as well as to reduce the amount of heat energy delivered to the subject.

Our current unit was manufactured by Kratos (USA) and utilizes a 2500-watt xenon arc source with filtration through a focusing lens, optional water cooler and dichroic mirror. Depending on the exact UV spectrum required, a variety of different UV filters can be employed in the lower housing unit. The present machine is air cooled, but when used previously with a 5000-W xenon arc lamp was water cooled.

Figures 1a, b show the spectral output derived with this unit. Other less powerful units utilize 150-W xenon arc lamps. One example of this is the Berger Solar Simulator. The main advantage of these smaller units is their portability, but the main disadvantage is that only small areas of skin irradiance are possible and therefore, they are really only suitable for pilot or smaller sunscreen studies. In comparison with the smaller units, the 1000–2500-W xenon arc machines can irradiate an area with relatively uniform skin irradiance of approximately 10 X 15 cm. With the xenon arc lamps, careful handling of the replacement lamps is most important as these lamps can explode and are a potential source of injury. In addition, the housing of the lamps have to be of sufficient strength to protect against such problems. The larger xenon arc-powdered units require cumbersome power supplies which take up considerable space and use significant amounts of energy.

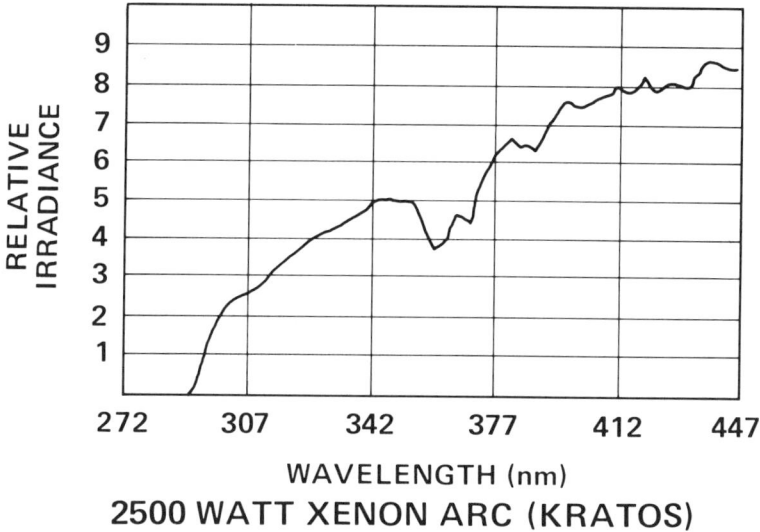

Figure 1a The spectral graph of a xenon arc solar simulator.

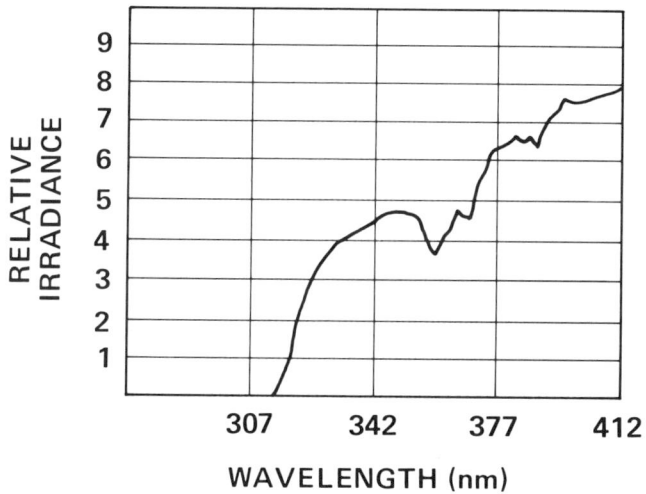

Figure 1b The spectrum of a xenon arc solar simulator filtered to provide UVA spectrum.

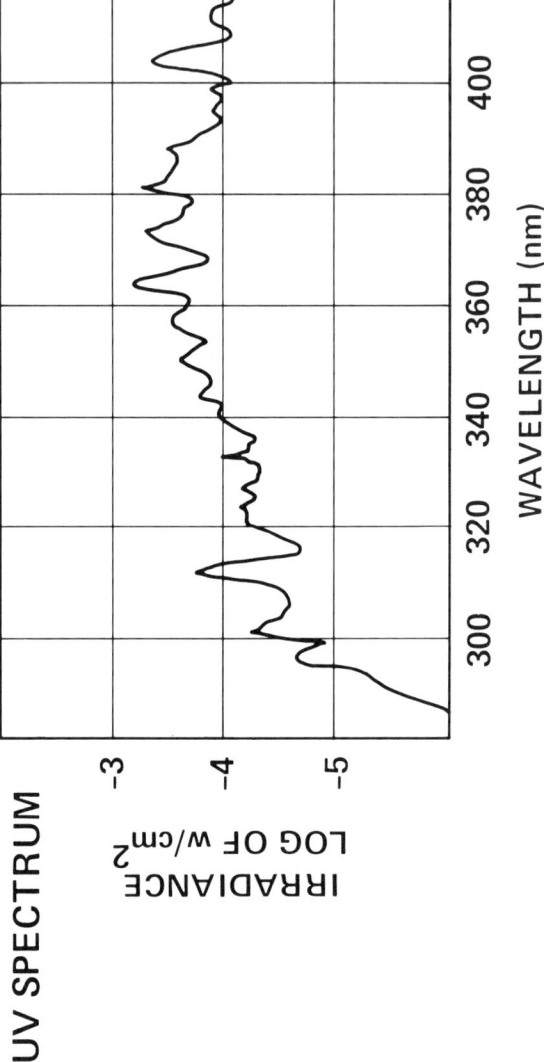

Figure 2   The spectrum of a high pressure metal halide simulator (Dermalight).

B. High-Pressure Metal Halide Sources

Mercury vapor lamps have been used for some years as ultraviolet sources, but their solar simulation has been considered poor because there are wide gaps between spectral lines in the ultraviolet range. The spectrum of the mercury vapor lamps can be improved using metal iodides to produce a more solar simulating spectrum (Fig. 2).

We recently had the opportunity to study the use of a high-pressure metal halide lamp as an appropriate ultraviolet source for sunscreen evaluation (2).

In a series of investigations, we compared the SPF numbers derived with a series of sunscreens comparing the filtered xenon arc lamp with the high-pressure metal halide simulator. Very similar SPF numbers were obtained utilizing these two machines (Table 4).

It would therefore seem feasable to use the high-pressure metal halide source as an alternative for sunscreen evaluation. One of the major advantages of this is that the machine is very portable and has a much higher energy output and larger skin irradiance area than does the 150-W xenon arc Solar Simulators.

C. Intermediate-Pressure Mercury Vapor Sources

The West German DIN system recommends the use of an Osram Vitalux Intermediate Pressure Mercury Vapor Source (5). This source is not solar simulating as it has a mercury vapor line spectrum. In comparison studies of predicted human SPF factors derived by utilizing the in vitro mouse epidermal assay, Sayre and Agin showed that the Osram Vitalux Lamp gave very similar predicted protection factors with most sunscreens when compared to the xenon arc solar simulator (6). Again, these studies suggest that there are realistic alternatives to using filtered xenon arc solar simulators. The Osram Vitalux unit is constructed using four bulbs arranged in a square grid, mounted at variable angles. The unit

Table 4 Comparison of SPFs Using Two Different Solar Simulators Mean SPF ± SD

	Metal halide SPF	Xenon arc SPF
Sunscreen		
Homosalate	3.8 ± 0.5	4.3 ± 0.5
A	15.0 ± 2.1	16.2 ± 1.6
B	9.4 ± 2.0	9.6 ± 1.7
C	15.6 ± 2.5	16.5 ± 1.5
D	16.2 ± 1.6	16.8 ± 1.6

Table 5 Comparison Between Xenon Arc, Metal Halide Simulators and Intermediate Pressure Mercury Vapor Sources

	Electrical power input (W)	UV per Watt	Simulation of solar spectrum	Lamp life (h)	Ease of operation	Cost of solar simulator	Running costs	Portability
Xenon arc	150–5000	Low	Excellent	1500	Complicated	High	High	150 W Yes 1000–5000 No
Metal halide	power 400–1000	High	Adequate	2000	Easy	Low	Low	Excellent
Intermediate pressure Mercury vapor	300	Low	Poor	2000	Easy	Low	Low	Possible

has to be suspended from the ceiling above the volunteer's back and hence, tends not to be as portable as for example the metal halide source.

D. Other Sources Used for SPF Testing

Other ultraviolet sources previously used have included flourescent sunlamp tubes. While these have the advantage of ease of use and of a consistent ultraviolet spectrum, their major disadvantage is they are not solar simulating (6) as they possess peak output at 313 nm with a lesser peak at 365. There is, therefore, relatively little UVA in relation to UVB, and in addition, these units do contain contaminant UVC.

Table 5 summarizes some differences between these UV sources.

E. Summary Comments on Ultraviolet Sources Used for Sunscreen Testing

Ideally, a close simulation of the solar spectrum is desirable for human SPF testing. This is clearly most simulated using filtered xenon arc sources. However, as discussed in this chapter, other units including a high-pressure metal halide simulator can be filtered to produce a relatively acceptable solar-simulating spectrum. The use of intermediate pressure mercury vapor units is also practical and is recommended in Germany. Comparison of the different types of alternative ultraviolet aparatus with the filtered xenon arc solar simulators have been conducted and show similar SPF numbers with some sunscreens.

V. OUTDOOR TESTING OF SUNSCREENS

The importance of outdoor testing has been stressed by some authorities (7) because of the need for evaluation of sunscreens in a setting more relevant to regular usage. In addition the volunteers are moving and therefore frictional removal of sunscreen is much more likely than in a static laboratory solar simulator environment. There is the additional important factor that sunlight contains larger amounts of infrared radiation than does solar simulator generated ultraviolet. In addition, there are other variables clearly relating to ambiant humidity, the possibility of sweating by volunteers hastening removal of some sunscreens. All of these factors make it very difficult to standardize outdoor sunscreen testing.

A more practical solution may be to intentionally vary indoor laboratory factors such as ambiant humidity, the amounts of infra-red radiance in the solar simulator spectrum and laboratory temperature. In this way a more controlled indoor reproducible evaluation of the sunscreens may be possible.

VI. WATER-RESISTANT AND WATERPROOF CLAIMS
OF SUNSCREEN PROTECTIVENESS

The FDA monograph (1) outlines the procedures required to evaluate sunscreens
in more rigorous conditions where the volunteers are exposed to different times
of water exposure following sunscreen application. These claims are divided into
two broad groups (See also Chap. 25).

A water-resistant property may be claimed by evaluating the subject after two
20-minute immersions with moderate activity in water. A waterproof claim requires four such immersions. Table 6 shows the types of protocols to be followed when evaluating either water-resistant or waterproof claims for sunscreens. In my laboratory, we have recently been evaluating a more controlled
series of procedures to test waterproofness and water resistance of sunscreen
products. These studies involve normal human volunteer forearm skin. A portable whirlpool bath was utilized with steady water movement provided by a
water agitator. The sunscreens were applied and the forearms immersed for the
appropriate amounts of time in the whirlpool tank.

Table 6 Protocols for Evaluating Sunscreen
Claims

Action	Time (min)
Water resistance claims protocol	
Apply sunscreen	0
In water	20
Out of water	40
In water	60
Out of water	80
Irradiate	100
Waterproof claims protocol	
Apply sunscreen	0
In water	20
Out of water	40
In water	60
Out of water	80
In water	100
Out of water	120
In water	140
Out of water	160
Irradiate	180

All erythema readings 24 h after irradiance.

Table 7 Waterproof Protocol Using Forearm Immersion in Whirlpool Tank
Control "static" SPF on contralateral nonimmersed forearm

Sun-screen	Nonwater-immersed control forearm SPF (mean)	Time (h) of water immersion SPF (mean)		
		1	2	3
A	32	25	23	20
B	30	–	–	21

For irradiance, the contralateral nonimmersed arm served for control non-water-immersed SPF numbers, whereas the immersed arm gave waterproof or resistant SPF numbers.

This has proved to be a reliable method. Table 7 shows preliminary results obtained with this method. With this equipment it is clearly practical to alter the water temperature, the degree of water agitation therefore simulating greater or lesser amounts of exercise. In addition, the degree of salinity can be altered to simulate either fresh water or sea water conditions. Few of these parameters have been studied in detail and it is planned to explore these in further detail with a further series of experiments using the solar simulator with this water immersion whirlpool unit.

VIII. RECENT TRENDS IN SUNSCREEN DEVELOPMENT

There are several recent important trends in sunscreen development. These include the increasing sun protection factor numbers, which have been mainly achieved using increasing amounts of sunscreen chemical. One concern has been a potential increased risk of irritancy and contact allergic sensitization reactions. Some sunscreens are now claiming SPF numbers of 50, and it remains to be seen whether there will be an increase in topical toxicity from these sunscreens (see Chap. 20).

Further areas of development include the development of micronized powders for use as physical reflecting sunscreens. This clearly will have great importance for patients with severely photosensitive skin diseases, but perhaps also as a means of reducing significant further UVA and infrared damage. There have also been suggestions that infrared radiance may be important as an additional cause particularly of sun induced skin aging (8-10). The current sunscreens absorb very poorly in infrared, but perhaps some of the new reflecting micronized powder sunscreens may afford better protection in this area of the solar spectrum.

The future potential risks of UVC irradiance should further ozone layer depletion occur in the atmosphere, may lead to the requirement to shift the absorption spectrum of sunscreens down to UVC. This, fortunately may be possible with some sunscreens, particularly with the PABA esters. It has additionally been shown that modification of the vehicle, for example, the use of more polar solvents may shift the absorption spectrum of several different sunscreens to the shorter wavelengths (11). Therefore, if there is more UVC irradiance reaching the earth's atmosphere in future years, it should be possible to modify the sunscreen to absorb at shorter ultraviolet wavelengths.

Clearly should such a change in the terrestrial solar spectrum occur then modification of ultraviolet sources used for phototesting would be required.

In summary, significant advances in sunscreen technology and testing have been achieved in recent years. Future developments are required, in particular, more efficient and cosmetically acceptable reflecting sunscreens that may have an enhanced photoprotection against UVA and infrared radiation and new ways of evaluating these different wavelengths and protection.

ACKNOWLEDGMENT

Some of the tables in this chapter were printed with permission from "Sunscreens and Phototesting," N.J. Lowe, D. Weingarten and M. Wortzman, in *Clinics in Dermatology*, Vol 6, pp. 40–49, 1988, Published by J.P. Lippincott.

REFERENCES

1. Sunscreen products for over-the-counter use. *Fed. Reg., 43*:28269 (1978).
2. Lowe, N. J., Weingarten, D., and Wortzman, M. Sunscreens and phototesting, *Clinics in Dermatology*, vol. 6 (W. Abramovits, ed.), J.B. Lippincott, Philadelphia (1988), pp. 40–49.
3. Stenberg, C. and Larko, O. Sunscreen application and its importance for the sun protection factor. *Arch. Dermatol., 121*:1400–1402 (1985).
4. Sayre, R. M. Sunscreen application: flawed study? (letter to the editor). *Arch. Dermatol., 122*:745–746 (1986).
5. Deutsches Institut fur Normung, Normenausschuss Litchttechnik, Berlin (1984).
6. Sayre, R. M. and Agin, P. P. Comparison of human sun protection factors to predicted protection factors using different lamp spectra. *J. Soc. Cosmet. Chem., 35*:439–445 (1984).
7. Pathak, M. Sunscreens: Topical and systemic approaches for protection of human skin against harmful effects of solar radiation. *J. Am. Acad. Dermatol., 7*:285–312 (1982).
8. Kligman, L. H. Intensification of ultraviolet induced dermal damage by infrared radiation. *Arch. Dermatol. Res.*, 227–229 (1982).

9. Freeman, R. G. and Knox, J. M. Influence of temperature on ultraviolet injury. *Arch. Dermatol., 89*:953–961 (1964).
10. Kligman, L. H. and Kligman, A. M. Reflections on heat. *Br. J. Dermatol., 110*:376–377 (1984).
11. Agradis-Palyompis, L., Nash, R., and Shaath, N. The effect of solvents on the ultraviolet absorbance of sunscreens. *J. Soc. Cosmet. Chem., 38*:209–221 (1987).

12
Substantivity and Water Resistance of Sunscreens

KAYS KAIDBEY   *University of Pennsylvania, Philadelphia, Pennsylvania*

A major achievement in the area of sunscreen research in recent years has been the development of highly substantive products which tend to resist washoff or removal by sweating. The main objective of this technology is to provide continuous photoprotection under varied and stressful environmental conditions, especially to those individuals who are excessively exposed to solar radiation such as outdoor workers, vacationers, swimmers, etc. On the whole, substantive products appear to be highly desirable among consumers, judging by the large number of currently marketed sunscreens with "waterproof" claims.

The ability of topically applied products to resist washoff is determined by several factors. The most important of these is the use of complex polymeric systems which apparently bind the active ingredient(s) on the surface of the skin, thus reducing the likelihood of dissolution into water. There are several such polymers being used at present and many others being investigated and developed. Polymer science is a highly specialized field which promises to affect every aspect of topical therapy.

Another major factor that can influence substantivity includes the design of the vehicle. Certain solvents can presumably enhance the penetration and deposition of sunscreen molecules into the stratum corneum, thus making them less accessible to water and rendering them less likely to be dissolved or removed by sweating, rubbing, or washing. Other aspects of the vehicle, such as viscosity may also influence substantivity. Viscous bases have better "adherence" properties to the stratum corneum compared, for example, to lotions. The physicochemical properties and behavior of the active sunscreen and its interaction with epidermal keratin molecules are also important. Octyldimethyl para amino benzoic acid (PABA), for example, is far more substantive than PABA, probably as a result of lower water solubility and better binding within the stratum corneum and hence is far better at resisting washoff (1). In contrast, PABA quickly penetrates the stratum corneum and diffuses into the dermis. Whatever is left on the surface of the skin is readily washed off (1).

Several tests have been recommended for evaluating the degree of substantivity. These include both in vitro and in vivo measurements. In vitro methods usually involve measurements of the amounts of sunscreens that can be "leached out" following a water immersion procedure or some other standardized exposure to water (2). A more accurate method involves the use of excised animal skin such as hairless mouse epidermis which is treated with sunscreens and then exposed to water in a bath at controlled temperatures for a certain time interval. Residual photoprotection can then be measured by forward-scattering spectrophotometry (3). Although these in vitro procedures have not gained widespread use, they are often employed in pilot studies to provide rough estimates of substantivity prior to human testing. In a preliminary investigation, Sayre et al. found that the in vitro prediction of post-washoff effectiveness using the mouse epidermis and forward scattering correlated well with substantivity measurements in vivo (3).

In the final analysis, in vivo human testing is the most acceptable and definitive method. Several procedures have been tried and these include the immersion of treated sites on the forearms in a water bath or a whirlpool for a measured period of time followed by exposure to UV to determine the degree of residual photoprotection (4,5). However, the most commonly used test for measuring the washoff resistance of sunscreens in this country is one that has been proposed by the FDA (6). In this procedure, a distinction is made between "water-resistant" and "waterproof" claims. The test itself is laborious and time consuming, but is straightforward in design. First, the sunscreen is applied at a topical dose of 2 mg/cm^2 to an area measuring at least 50 cm^2 over the midback and the static SPF is determined. Following that, the test product is reapplied to an adjoining test site and after a drying period of about 15–20 minutes, the subjects are then supposed to engage in an "activity in the water" for a 20-minute interval in an indoor swimming pool. The word "activity" in the water rather than swimming is used presumably because the majority of individuals may not be able to swim for the entire duration of the test. After a rest period of 20 minutes, there follows another 20-minute interval of water exposure followed in turn by air drying without toweling and then exposure to the solar simulator. Thus, for water resistance testing, a total of 40 minutes in the water is specified whereas for a waterproof claim, the total duration in the water is extended to 80 minutes, which again is achieved through 20-minute intervals in the water, separated by 20-minute rest periods. The postbathing SPF is then determined and if the mean value falls in the same product category designation as that before bathing, a water-resistance or waterproof claim is allowed. It is generally accepted that this is a more severe test than the sweating test and hence water-resistant or waterproof products can be presumed to be sweat resistant as well. Indoor testing is recommended in order to limit exposure to solar UV.

There are several aspects of this test that need to be addressed in more detail. It is clear that the use of fresh rather than salt water is appropriate and adds to the severity of the test since salt or sea water should have a lower dissolving effect because of the salt content ($\sim$3%). We have found that the degree of chlorination does not have a perceptible or measurable effect on the post washoff SPF. Several years ago, in an effort to standardize the washoff test further and make it more uniform, we determined post-washoff SPFs using an indoor water-tank similar to a whirlpool (7). The tank was equipped with a pump which generated a constant "background" current. This set-up was thought to provide a more uniform and constant exposure to water than swimming or casual activity in a swimming pool. The exposure intervals in the water, punctuated by 20-minute rest periods, were otherwise as recommended in the FDA monograph. The post-washoff SPFs of several products were determined in the whirlpool and compared to values obtained in a swimming pool. Table 1 shows that the results were in general similar. Subsequent comparisons made on different occasions in larger panels of subjects have reconfirmed that original finding. We have concluded on the basis of these comparisons that the whirlpool method is far more convenient and provides a more uniform and probably more stringent exposure to water than the swimming pool test, in view of the constant and more powerful current that can be generated in such a setup. Another factor that can influence the post-washoff SPF is the water temperature. As a result of a series of tests that were conducted with certain products at different water

Table 1 Comparison of Post-Wash-off SPFs Obtained in a Laboratory Whirlpool and an Indoor Swimming Pool

Sunscreen	Static SPF	Post-washoff SPF	Post-swimming SPF
A. Octyldimethyl PABA	8.4 ± 1.6	4.0 ± 1.2	3.6 ± 0.8
B. Octyldimethyl PABA	4.5 ± 0.9	4.0 ± 1.2	4.6 ± 1.6
C. Octyldimethyl PABA Oxybenzone	11.8 ± 2.0	4.3 ± 1.8	4.2 ± 1.0
D. Octyldimethyl PABA Oxybenzone	21.0 ± 1.1	18.1 ± 1.5	>19.0

Source: Reproduced with permission from the Journal of the American Academy of Dermatology, the C.F. Mosby Company, St. Louis, Missouri.

temperatures, it was possible in retrospect to compare the post-washoff SPFs under the different temperature conditions. An example of such a comparison is shown in Table 2. The results suggest that at the higher temperature range, the post-washoff SPF tends to be lower. Because of such differences, it is important to maintain a careful control over the water temperature during the procedure. In the FDA monograph, the suggested temperature range (21–32°C) is probably too broad and should be narrowed down for reproducibility. We currently maintain the whirlpool water temperature between 29 and 30°C.

During the past 10 years, this laboratory has generated a considerable amount of data on the post-washoff SPF and substantivity of sunscreen products. It has become very clear that products which contain similar active ingredients at equivalent or identical concentrations differ greatly in their degree of photoprotection following a washoff test. This again underscores the important role of the vehicle on substantivity. The effect of the vehicle on substantivity in general is illustrated by the data in Table 3. It can be seen that, contrary to earlier assertions, PABA itself is not substantive and is washedoff during a 40-minute exposure to water. We had previously demonstrated that the vehicle can also markedly influence the static SPF (7), but this factor becomes even more crucial in providing resistance to washoff. Certain products which are water resistant also prove to be waterproof and hence seem to lose little of their effectiveness following the extended washoff procedure (Table 4).

Recently, several products with very high SPFs ranging from 30 to 50 have appeared with waterproof claims. It is not clear whether a product with a post-washoff SPF of 50 for example is really necessary or required or whether these numbers reflect static values rather than post-washoff values. Consequently, we have evaluated the post wash-off SPF of some of these products using the indoor whirlpool method as described previously at a temperature of 30°C. The mean SPFs are shown in Table 5. Only three of the eight tested products had a post-washoff waterproof SPF which was accurately reflected on the label.

There remains several unanswered questions about the washoff test. Even under rigorously controlled laboratory conditions, variability can be a major

Table 2 Mean Post-Washoff SPFs (±SD) of Three Sunscreens Obtained at Different Temperature Ranges

Sunscreen	Water temperature 32–35°C	Water temperature 24–27°C
A	14.2 ± 1.0	17.7 ± 1.1
B	16.7 ± 0.9	20.3 ± 1.2
C	14.4 ± 1.3	> 18.7

Table 3 Influence of Vehicle on Substantivity of Various Sunscreen Preparations (n=10)

Sunscreen	Static SPF	Post-washoff[a] SPF
A. 5% PABA	8.0 ± 0.9	1.2 ± 0.4
B. 10% Sulisobenzone	10.1 ± 2.1	1.3 ± 0.2
C. 8.0% Octyldimethyl PABA	8.4 ± 1.6	4.03 ± 0.1
D. 5.5% Octyldimethyl PABA 3.0% Oxybenzone	11.8 ± 2.0	4.3 ± 1.8
E. 3.3% Octyldimethyl PABA	4.5 ± 0.9	4.0 ± 1.2
F. 8% Octyldimethyl PABA 3% Oxybenzone	21.0 ± 1.1	18.1 ± 1.5

[a]Indoor water tank (water-resistance test).
Source: Reproduced with permission from the American Academy of Dermatology, the C.V. Mosby Company, St. Louis, Missouri.

Table 4 A Comparison of Post-Washoff SPFs of Two Sunscreens Following a Water Resistance and a Waterproof Test

Sunscreen	40-Min washoff	80-Min washoff
A	36.0 ± 4.1	29.3 ± 8.6
B	36.1 ± 5.8	35.7 ± 4.7
C	21.0 ± 2.3	22.0 ± 3.6

Table 5 Post-washoff (Waterproof) SPFs of Several Marketed High-Efficacy Waterproof Sunscreens

Sunscreen (waterproof label)	Post-washoff SPF ± SD	N
A (SPF 29)	29.2 ± 4.3	21
B (SPF 30)	29.9 ± 2.6	10
C (SPF 30)	23.3 ± 3.6	11
D (SPF 30)	22.8 ± 4.4	10
E (SPF 30)	22.1 ± 6.2	11
F (SPF 39)	39.2 ± 2.5	20
G (SPF 40)	31.9 ± 4.4	10
H (SPF 50)	31.7 ± 7.1	10

difficulty. Thus in every panel, we have usually encountered one or more individuals in whom an otherwise effective product appears to have washed off, occasionally resulting in a painful sunburn in the test sites. The reason(s) for this is not known, nor is it clear what or how to deal with these values. In preliminary studies, where the testing was repeated in these same individuals, the test products did produce the expected degree of protection. Hence, it appears likely that in these cases, the test sites were accidentally rubbed or touched by clothing or other articles such as towels. Another factor which has received little attention is reproducibility of the test data. Clearly, much more work needs to be done to clarify these issues.

REFERENCES

1. Blank, I. H., Ornellas, L., Anderson, R. R., Mosher, D. B., and Parrish, J. A. Observations on the substantivity of sunscreens. Abstract presented at the Seventh Annual Meeting of the American Society of Photobiology, June, Asilomar, Pacific Grove, CA (1979).
2. Morasso, M. I., Thielemann, A. M., Pinto, C., Figueroa, M., and Arancibia, A. In vitro and in vivo study of the substantivity of p-aminobenzoic acid and two of its esters. *J. Soc. Cosmet. Chem., 36*:355 (1985).
3. Sayre, R. M., PohAgin, P., Desrochers, D. L., and Marlowe, E. Sunscreen testing methods: In vitro predictions of effectiveness. *J. Soc. Cosmet. Chem., 31*:133 (1980).
4. Greiter, F., Bilek, P., Doskoczil, S., Washuttl, J., and Wurst, F. Methods for water resistance testing of sun protection products. *Int. J. Cosmet. Sci., 1*: 147 (1979).
5. Sayre, R. M., Marlowe, E., PohAgin, P., LeVee, G. J., and Rosenberg, W. Performance of six sunscreen formulations on human skin. *Arch. Dermatol., 115*:46 (1979).
6. Department of Health, Education and Welfare, U.S. F.D.A. Sunscreen drug products for over-the-counter human drugs. *Fed. Reg., 43*:38206 (1978).
7. Kaidbey, K. H. and Kligman, A. M. An appraisal of the efficacy and substantivity of the new high-potency sunscreens. *J. Am. Acad. Dermatol., 4*:566 (1981).

13

Sunscreens: Effects of Amounts of Application of Sun Protection Factors

ANNETTE GOTTLIEB *UCLA School of Medicine, Los Angeles, California*

TERESA D. BOURGET *Skin Research Foundation of California, Santa Monica, California*

NICHOLAS J. LOWE *Skin Research Foundation of California, Santa Monica, California, and UCLA School of Medicine, Los Angeles, California*

I. OVERVIEW

There has been controversy about the amount of sunscreen applied by individuals. At least one previous study of a group of volunteers suggested that approximately 1 mg/cm² was the average application by a participant. This contrasted with the amount (2 mg/cm²) routinely advised for routine human evaluation of sun protection factors in the USA. We have re-evaluated different sunscreen formulations: a gel, an alcoholic lotion, a creamy lotion, and a cream used by a group of volunteers. We found the mean application amount to be 1.3 mg/cm² with the gel applied in a slightly greater thickness overall at 1.7 mg/cm². Sun protection factor (SPF) studies were then performed using a filtered xenon arc solar simulator and five different sunscreens.

Four of the sunscreens showed no significant reduction of SPF using sunscreen application of 1.3 mg/cm² compared with 2.0 mg/cm². However, one sunscreen with an SPF of 29 at 2.0 mg/cm² did show a significant decrease in protection at lower application amounts.

II. EVALUATING THE APPROPRIATE AMOUNT OF SUNSCREEN USAGE

Sunscreen use is now felt to be established as an important means of reducing the risks of photocarcinogenesis (1) and photoaging (2). The Food and Drug Administration (FDA) developed guidelines in 1978 for evaluating the protectiveness of a sunscreen (3). This monograph recommended that sunscreens be delivered at 2 mg or 2 μl/cm^2 amounts. Most of the claimed sun protection factor (SPF) numbers of sunscreens appropriately evaluated in the United States have therefore been determined using this quantity of sunscreen.

A previous study reported that sunscreens may in fact be delivered at much smaller amounts of approximately 1 mg/cm^2, resulting in a lower SPF (4). This particular investigation was subsequently criticized (5) for some important reasons. Only a small sample of sunscreen was supplied (albeit per each area of the body), which may have artificially restricted the quantity of sunscreen applied. (A study by Lynfield and Schechter (6), found that individuals will use less than half the amount of topical medication supplied in a small tube compared with that in a large jar.) Another problem was that a nonsolar-simulating source was used which may have resulted in relatively low SPF numbers. Also, the products used in the study are not available in the United States.

We therefore undertook a study to further investigate average amounts of sunscreens applied by individuals. In addition, we have determined the protection factors of several different sunscreens using the average amount applied by our volunteers. These SPF values have been compared with values for the same sunscreens applied at 2.0 and 1.0 mg/cm^2.

III. MATERIALS AND METHODS

For the application density studies, the following four sunscreen preparations were used:

Clear Gel. Padimate O (octyl dimethyl PABA), glyceryl PABA, with: alcohol (55%), water, PEG-6, carbomer-940, and hydroxyethylcellulose

Clear Lotion. 5% Amino benzoic acid (PABA), 5% padimate O (octyl dimethyl PABA), 3% oxybenzone, 58% SD alcohol 40

Creamy Lotion. Octyl methoxycinnamate, oxybenzone, octyl salicylate

Cream. 7% Ethylhexyl P-methoxycinnamate, 4% oxybenzone, 2% titanium dioxide

A. Evaluation of Sunscreen Application Amounts

After informed consent was obtained, 20 healthy volunteers (17 women and three men) were randomly divided into four groups in which the individuals were asked to apply a particular kind of sunscreen as follows: (1) creamy lotion, (2) clear lotion, (3) clear gel, (4) cream. The active ingredients in the different sunscreens are described above. The sunscreens were kept in their individual large-sized bottles as they would appear if bought in a store. The individuals were instructed to apply a particular sunscreen, using as much as they normally would if they were going to the beach to six separate regions of the body: head and neck, chest, back, arms, thighs, and lower legs. Subjects wore sterile plastic gloves and applied the desired amount of sunscreen to one region at a time under the observation of one of the investigators. By weighing the sunscreen bottle and the gloves before and after each application and subtracting, the amount used per body region was determined, taking into account any residual sunscreen left on the hands. The height and weight of each volunteer was obtained and the body surface area was calculated using a nomogram (7). The specific surface area for each body region was calculated using a modification of the "rule of 9's" for estimating burn injuries (8). In this way, we were able to determine the average layer thicknesses of four different sunscreens applied to various locations of the body.

B. Evaluation of Sun Protection Factors

For the studies of application densities, a filtered xenon arc solar simulator was used. Five sunscreens were used which had manufacturer-determined SPFs of 4, 8, 10, 15, and 29, respectively. (The sunscreen with the SPF of 4 was a standard formulation provided by the FDA which was used as a control.) Controls were normal healthy volunteers who had skin types 1 or 2, based upon their history of skin responses to prior sun exposure (skin type 1 sunburns and does not tan, skin type 2 sunburns and tans slightly). Lower back or buttock skin, which was not previously sun exposed was utilized for the studies. Informed consent was obtained after the procedure was fully explained.

On the first study day, the minimal erythema dose (MED) was determined for each volunteer by irradiating the unprotected skin with 25% increments of ultraviolet light around the anticipated MED for that skin type. The MED was the shortest light exposure at which erythema was observed 24 hours later and below which no visible change was noted. Using a measuring micrometer syringe, sunscreens were carefully applied to achieve a uniform layer using a micropipette at 2.0, 1.3, and 1.0 $\mu l/cm^2$ over a precut template 1 × 6 cm with square holes 1 cm^2 placed on the skin. These sites were irradiated using a series of ultraviolet doses around the anticipated MED of the protected skin, as detailed by the recommended procedures in the FDA sunscreen monograph (3). A 2500 W filtered xenon arc solar simulator (Kratos) was used for irradiance. The skin was observed 24 hours later and the actual SPF was determined by dividing the MED of the protected skin by that of the unprotected skin. In this way, the actual

SPFs of five different sunscreens applied in three different layer thicknesses were determined.

IV. RESULTS

A. Amounts of Sunscreen Applied

There was variation in the amounts of sunscreen applied (Table 1) among the different body regions.

   Overall, the average amount of sunscreen applied was 1.3 mg/cm^2. In general, the gel was applied at a greater density (average amount = 1.7 mg/cm^2) than the other vehicles in all areas of the body except for the back.

B. Sun Protection Factors

There was no significant change in SPF for four of the tested sunscreens with applied amounts of 1.0 and 1.3 μl/cm^2 compared with 2.0 μl/cm^2. However, the fifth sunscreen (with a manufacturer-determined SPF of 29) did show a significant decrease in SPF both at 1.0 and at 1.3 μl/cm^2. The results are summarized in Table 2.

Table 1   Average Amount of Sunscreen Applied to Various Regions of the Body (mg/cm^2) (mean ± SD)

Sunscreen	Head and neck (n = 5)	Chest (n = 5)	Back (n = 5)	Arms (n = 5)	Thighs (n = 5)	Lower legs (n = 5)
Creamy lotion	1.85 ± 0.66	1.10 ± 0.27	0.95 ± 0.40	1.28 ± 0.45	1.16 ± 0.31	1.11 ± 0.41
Alcoholic lotion	1.54 ± 0.73	1.16 ± 0.78	1.45 ± 0.95	1.27 ± 0.56	1.07 ± 0.26	1.28 ± 0.36
Gel	2.23 ± 1.01	1.49 ± 0.50	1.26 ± 0.40	1.76 ± 0.64	1.97 ± 0.48	1.59 ± 0.85
Cream	1.03 ± 0.42	1.17 ± 0.58	0.93 ± 0.64	1.05 ± 0.53	1.38 ± 0.82	0.94 ± 0.77

Table 2 Sun Protection Factors for Five Sunscreens Applied in Three Different Amounts (mean ± SD)

Amount applied (μl/cm^2)	Sunscreens[a]				
	A	B	C	D	E
2.0	4.0 ± 0.37 (n = 14)	8.7 ± 1.22 (n = 14)	11.0 ± 1.74 (n = 14)	16.0 ± 1.76 (n = 14)	29.0 ± 1.73 (n = 5)
1.3	4.2 ± 0.48 (n = 15)	8.0 ± 1.03 (n = 15)	11.1 ± 1.41 (n = 15)	14.8 ± 1.80 (n = 15)	25.0 ± 2.12[b] (n = 5)
1.0	4.3 ± 0.44 (n = 5)	7.8 ± 0.44 (n = 5)	10.0 ± 1.41 (n = 5)	14.4 ± 1.34 (n = 5)	17.4 ± 1.34[b] (n = 5)

[a]Manufacturer-determined SPFs are as follows: A=SPF 4; B=SPF 8; C=SPF 10; D=SPF 15; E=SPF 29.
[b]The mean SPF value is statistically different from the mean SPF for the same sunscreen applied at 2.0 μl/cm^2 ($p < 0.05$).

V. DISCUSSION

The present study was undertaken to determine the average amount of sunscreen applied by most individuals, and to evaluate the subsequent effect on sun protection factors. We found the average sunscreen application amount to be 1.3 mg/cm^2, which was close to 1 mg/cm^2 found in a previous study by Stenberg and Larko (4). The gel was applied in a slightly greater amount as compared to the other vehicles (mean = 1.7 mg/cm^2) in all areas of the body except for the back. (Since the back is the most difficult area to reach, it is also probably the most unreliable area with regard to application.) Otherwise, the varying consistencies of the different sunscreens did not appear to play a role in application density, which differs from the findings of Stenberg and Larko. It is likely that in routine use even lower amounts than those documented in this study may actually be delivered to the skin. This may occur when sunscreen is applied hurriedly or with application to both hairy skin and to areas of the body which are difficult to reach.

In the United States, to obtain claimed SPF values, a sunscreen amount of 2 mg/cm^2 or 2 μl/cm^2 is recommended (3). Our results, in contrast to those of Stenberg and Larko (4), suggest that individuals may apply less than the 2 mg/cm^2 quantity without diminishing the SPF value, at least with regard to lower SPF sunscreens. It is noteworthy that an SPF 29 sunscreen retained an SPF of 25 with 1.3 μl/cm^2 and 17.4 with 1.0 μl/cm^2; this suggests that the use of high

SPF sunscreens (greater than 15) may still offer maximal protection even if the sunscreen is applied in less than optimum quantities.

These results are not in agreement with those of Stenberg and Larko (4) who found that 1 mg/cm^2 gave only 50% of the protection achieved with the 2 mg/cm^2 application. This may be due to the different methods employed: They used a glass rod to apply a defined amount of sunscreen to a 10 X 30 cm area. We used a micropipette to apply microliter amounts to 1 cm^2 areas. Perhaps, by dealing with much smaller skin areas we were able to achieve more uniform layers and thus retain more sunscreen protection.

We were careful to incorporate the suggestions of Sayre (5) including the use of a filtered xenon arc solar simulator (as stipulated in the current FDA monograph on evaluation of sunscreens), supplying large standardized purchased sunscreen containers to the volunteers, and using products that are available in the United States. Our results suggest that, as in other countries such as Germany (9), a more appropriate sunscreen delivery amount for phototesting should be lower than 2 μl/cm^2. Other studies are needed to decide if this amount should be 1.5 μl/cm^2 as used in the West Germany Deutsches Institut für Normung (DIN) investigations.

REFERENCES

1. Parrish, J. A., et al. UV-A; *Biological Effects of Ultraviolet Radiation with Emphasis on Human Responses to Longwave Ultraviolet*, Plenum Press, New York (1978).
2. Kligman, L. H. and Kligman, A. M. The nature of photoaging: its prevention and repair. *Photodermatology*, *3*:215–227 (1986).
3. Department of Health, Education and Welfare. U.S.: Sunscreen drug products for over-the-counter human use. *Fed. Reg.*, *43*:38206–38269 (1978).
4. Stenberg, C. and Larko, O. Sunscreen application and its importance for the sun protection factor. *Arch. Dermatol.*, *121*:1400–1402 (1985).
5. Sayre, R. M. Sunscreen application: flawed study? (Lett.). *Arch. Dermatol.*, *122*:745–746 (1986).
6. Lynfield, Y. L. and Schechter, S. Choosing and using a vehicle. *J. Am. Acad. Dermatol.*, *10*:55–59 (1984).
7. Goraef, J. W. and Cone, T. E. Jr. (eds.). *Manual of Pediatric Therapeutics*, 3rd ed., Little, Brown and Co., Boston (1985).
8. *Plastic and Reconstructive Surgery – Essentials for Students*, Plastic Surgery Educational Foundation, Chicago (1986), p. 85.
9. Martini, M. C. Comparison des méthodes de détermination des SPF. *Int. J. Cosmet. Sci.*, *8*:215–224 (1986).

14
UVA Photoprotection

NICHOLAS J. LOWE *Skin Research Foundation of California, Santa Monica, California, and UCLA School of Medicine, Los Angeles, California*

I. UVA EFFECTS ON THE SKIN

It is a well established finding that ultraviolet radiation causes damage to the skin; damage which results in both precancerous and cancerous skin lesions as well as enhancement of normal skin aging.

The shorter more energetic UVB wavelengths are primarily absorbed in the epidermis and upper parts of the dermis. The longer UVA wavelengths penetrate to the lower dermis. Recently, attention has been directed at the effects of UVA on the dermis, in particular its possible ability to enhance skin aging. It has also been suggested, from animal studies (1), that UVA is capable of augmenting the photocarcinogenic effects of UVB. In addition, UVA has also been shown capable, in human skin, of enhancing UVB-induced erythema (2). UVA in sufficient amounts will also effect direct release of a variety of vasoactive mediators responsible for skin erythema and inflammatory reactions (3).

UVB intensity varies considerably with season and geographic location. However, in general, the intensity of UVA irradiation is more consistent than UVB.

The approximate minimal erythema doses (MED) for a skin type I individual who burns readily and tans minimally in sunlight for UVB is 0.03 J/cm^2. The approximate UVA-induced minimal erythema dose for the skin type I individual is 30 J/cm^2. Therefore, UVA is considerably less photoactive for erythema induction in a nonphotosensitized individual than UVB.

A. UVA-Induced Photosensitization

UVA is extremely important, as the wavelengths that produce photosensitivity in individuals taking certain photosensitizing drugs or having photosensitizing diseases are within the UVA spectrum.

In addition, there are several photosensitivity diseases that have their action spectra either completely or partially within UVA. Table 1 lists some of those diseases. Some of these diseases will now be discussed briefly.

B. Polymorphous Light Eruption

Polymorphous light eruption is a common skin eruption and occurs in suscepti-ble individuals at the start of the summer season or when they visit a geographi-cal area with higher solar radiation than they usually experience. The skin lesions take several different forms, as implied by the term polymorphous. Classically, the eruption consists of pruritic papules, macules, plaques, or confluent ery-thema. A variant form of this manifests as multiple pruritic erythemetous papules and vesicles termed papulovesicular light eruption.

Typically the lesions and symptoms develop 1 to 2 days after sun exposure. In some cases, the eruption gradually improves on continued sun exposure and tolerance may be induced by careful delivery of either UVB irradiation or psoralen plus UVA (PUVA) therapy (4).

Management usually involves avoiding excessive sun exposure or gradually increasing sun exposure to induce tolerance. The use of sunscreens and topical corticosteroids are sometimes helpful. A problem for many people suffering from polymorphous light eruption is that the action spectrum of their disease extends into the longer UVA wavelengths (5). Unfortunately, many of the cur-rent sunscreens only partially protect in these UVA wavelengths and are poorly effective at protecting against polymorphous light eruption (5,6).

Table 1 Photosensitivity Diseases

Diseases that are either initiated or exacerbated by ex-posure to UV wave-lengths include:

Polymorphous light eruption (PMLE) (290–365 nm)
Chronic actinic dermatitis (290–360 nm)
Actinic reticuloid (290–540 nm)
Lupus erythematosus (290–330 nm)
Solar urticaria (290–515 nm)
Persistent light reaction (290–400 nm)
Xeroderma pigmentosum (290–340 nm)

In addition to topical sunscreens, some individuals occasionally can control these eruptions with systemic antimalarial therapy or oral beta carotene. In Europe, thalidamide has been used as an effective treatment for more severe cases of polymorphous light eruption in males and older women. This condition therefore requires more efficient UVA sunscreening chemicals.

C. Chronic Actinic Dermatitis

Chronic actinic dermatitis and actinic reticuloid are two ends of a spectrum of photosensitivity diseases. Commonly, the skin eruption starts initially on exposed skin and consists of erythematous papules and plaques, later progressing to chronic infiltrated skin lesions. The patients are exquisitely photosensitive to a wide range of wavelengths, including UVA. It is considered that chronic actinic dermatitis is the less severe end of the clinical spectrum with actinic recticuloid being the more severe. The histology of actinic reticuloid skin lesions resembles that of a cutaneous T-cell lymphoma. Acurate phototesting is important in the investigation of these conditions as it may be necessary to advise different types of photoprotection depending on the range of ultraviolet responsible for the induction of the disease.

D. Solar Urticaria

This rare condition is characterized by the rapid onset of itching with subsequent urticaria and erythema within minutes after sun or ultraviolet exposure. The wavelength responsible for different types of solar urticaria varies considerably, as can be seen from Table 1. Skin lesions are usually transient and last less than 24 hours. Treatment has been largely unsatisfactory. Again, careful phototesting and the identification of the responsible wavelengths are important so that appropriate advice can be given as to the value of different sunscreens. UVA-absorbing as well as UVB-absorbing sunscreens are important in the management of some patients with this condition.

E. Lupus Erythematosis

Photosensitivity to UVB radiation is usually important in patients with cutaneous lupus erythematosis. In addition, however, some patients do react within UVA and there have been reports of UVA suntanning establishments inducing lesions in a patient with systemic lupus erythematosus.

Rigorous protection against sunlight is required, and this would include the use of UVB- as well as UVA-absorbing sunscreens.

F. Photoallergic and Phototoxic Reactions

A considerable number of different drugs are available, which are capable of producing photosensitivity eruptions. Most of the responsible wavelengths are in UVA (Table 2).

G. Photoallergic Reactions

Photoallergic reactions are less common than phototoxic reactions and occur where there has been a combination of previous exposure to the drug with sufficient exposure to ultraviolet radiation to produce photosensitization. Subsequent exposure then produces the clinical lesions. Important causes of photoallergic reactions include halogenated salicylanilides, musk ambrette, and fentichlor. Diagnosis is confirmed by careful photopatch testing. The action spectra for most photoallergic reactions are in the UVA wavelengths. Drug-induced photoallergic reactions may also occur, and some potential photoallergic drugs include sulfonamides, thiazide diuretics, and nonsteroidal anti-inflammatory agents. It is noted that these drugs may also produce phototoxic reactions. It is sometimes possible to confirm the photoallergic drug or chemical by careful phototesting and photopatch testing. Subsequent withdrawal of that drug and the use of broad-spectrum sunscreens and sun avoidance is clearly very important.

Some patients, unfortunately, become persistent light reactors following photoallergic reactions. This condition may persist long after the drug or chemical is withdrawn from their environment and, presumably, represents a persistent photoimmunological abnormality.

Table 2 Drugs and Wavelengths of Light Responsible for Photosensitivity Reactions

Drug	Wavelength range (nm)
8-Methoxypsoralen	320–400
Coal tar	340–430
Tetracycline	320–400
Piroxicam	320–400
Hydrochlorothiazide	320–400
Chlorpromazine	320–400
Griseofulvin	320–400
Amiodarone	290–400

H. Phototoxic Reactions

Phototoxic reactions occur in all persons exposed to a phototoxic agent providing sufficient agent and ultraviolet radiation are available to produce the skin reaction. 8-Methoxypsoralen (used in the therapy of psoriasis, vitiligo, and cutaneous lymphoma) produces phototoxic reactions if excessive amounts of UVA are delivered. Patients taking sulfonamide antibiotics, tetracyclines, thiazide diuretics, nonsteroidal anti-inflammatory agents such as piroxicam, phenothiazines, and amiodarone may suffer phototoxic reactions (Table 2).

Because the action spectra for most phototoxic reactions lie within UVA, there is a case to be made for the routine use of UVA-absorbing sunscreens in the management of patients taking potential phototoxic drugs.

II. UVA-ABSORBING SUNSCREENS

There are currently four principal sunscreening chemicals allowed by the food and drug administration (FDA). These are: oxybenzone, sulisobenzone, dioxybenzone, and menthyl anthranilate (Table 3).

A newer UVA-absorbing sunscreen chemical has recently been approved by the FDA. This is butyl methoxydibenzoylmethane, also known as Parsol 1789.

Most of these UVA-absorbing chemicals are poorly effective in absorbing UVB wavelengths. Therefore, for a sunscreen to possess broad-spectrum UVB and UVA absorption the UVA screens are usually combined with UVB absorbers such as octyldimethyl PABA or one of the cinnamates. The physical sunblock also contributes to UVA absorption.

III. EVALUATION OF UV-ABSORBING SUNSCREENING CHEMICALS

A. Selection of UV Sources

As with the evaluation of sun protection factor (SPF) (7) the selection of UV-emitting sources is of critical importance for the evaluation of UVA photoprotection. Sources such as flourescent sunlamp tubes or OSRAM vitalux sources are clearly inappropriate for UVA studies as they emit very poorly in UVA. The solar spectrum contains large amounts of UVA wavelengths in comparison to UVB and so should experimental UV sources used. Suitable UVA sources include appropriately filtered xenon arc solar simulators. Using different filters, it is possible to select a relatively solar-simulating profile of UVA emission. In this laboratory, we have used a xenon arc source filtered with either mylar or with a WG-345 filter to produce a UVA spectrum (8).

Table 3   FDA-OTC Panel Category I Approved Sunscreens and Concentrations

	Approved %
1. Chemical	
UVA Absorbers	
Oxybensone	2–6
Sulisobenzone	5–10
Dioxybenzone	3
menthyl anthranilate	3.5–5
UVB Absorbers	
Amino benzoic acid	5–15
Amyl dimethyl PABA	1–5
2-Ethoxyethyl *p*-methoxy cinnamate	1–3
Diethanolamine *p*-methoxy cinnamate	8–10
Digalloyl trioleate	2–5
Ethyl 4-*bis* (hydroxypropyl) aminobenzoate	1–5
2-Ethylhexyl-2-cyano-3,3-diphenylacrylate	7–10
Ethylhexyl *p*-methoxy cinnamate	2–7.5
2-Ethylhexyl salicylate	3–5
Glyceryl aminobenzoate	2–3
Homomenthyl salicylate	4–15
Lawsone with dihydroxyacetone	0.25 with 3
Octyl dimethyl PABA	1.4–8
2-Phenylbenzimidazole-5-sulfonic acid	1.4
Triethanolamine salicylate	5–12
2. Physical	
Red petrolatum	30–100
Titanium dioxide	2–25

An alternative and convenient source is an appropriately filtered high pressure metal halide source with emitting between 315 and 400 nm. Again such a source has a UV emission profile similar to that of the solar spectrum (9).

Another source that has been utilized for UVA photoprotection is a "Mutzhas lamp" (10). A criticism of the spectrum of that lamp is that its lower wavelength emission starts at about 340 nm. Therefore, it does not contain the important shorter UVA wavelengths that are probably responsible for significant photobiological effects of UVA. In addition, the peak action spectra for a variety of phototoxic reactions and photoallergic reactions lie within the shorter UVA wavelengths.

Both the filtered xenon arc solar simulator and high-pressure metal halide simulator emit throughout the UVA spectrum and are ideal sources for assessment of UVA-induced effects on the skin (9,10).

B. UVA-Induced Erythema as a Means of Evaluating Sunscreens

Classical sun protection factor (SPF testing) for UVA sunscreening chemicals has been difficult because large amounts of UVA are required to produce skin erythema even in fair-skinned individuals. The ultraviolet output of traditional solar simulators and ultraviolet sources has been too low to make this form of evaluation of UVA protection practical. For testing of a UVA protection factor of 3-4, the volunteer subject would have to be exposed to approximately 100-120 J/cm^2 of UVA. With most UV sources, extremely long irradiance times are required.

There have been attempts recently to use higher intensity UVA sources (11). These studies found that erythema alone produced by a high-intensity UVA source was poorly visualized. Some of the practical difficulties may involve the induction of erythema due to heating of the skin by the long irradiance time required. In addition, the pigmentation response from ultraviolet may obscure the UVA-induced erythema.

It is possible that higher intensity UVA-emitting sources could be developed which would be capable of producing shorter irradiance times. Further studies recently in this area of research (see Chap. 31).

C. UVA-Induced Immediate Pigmentation as a Means of Evaluating UVA Sunscreens

It is possible to produce immediate pigment darkening from UVA irradiation. This observation has been used as means of evaluating UVA sunscreens (11,12). A variety of sunscreens were evaluated using this technique. Relatively low "UVA protection factors" were obtained for these sunscreens and it is not likely that this will prove to be a satisfactory means of evaluating UVA protection probably because the action spectra for immediate pigment darkening is very broad and covers wavelengths other than UVA. The immediate pigmentation was evaluated 10 minutes following irradiation. In addition, delayed tanning responses were also evaluated in the same subjects at 24 hours (12).

D. UVA-Induced Photosensitization as a Means of Evaluating UVA Photoprotection

In our laboratory, we have used topical methoxalen photosensitization in healthy volunteers to determine UVA photoprotection factors with a variety of UVA sunscreening agents (8). These studies were initially conducted using a window glass filtered xenon arc solar simulator. The results were subsequently confirmed out of doors using mylar filtered sunlight to produce UVA irradiance (8). The indoor source and outdoor filtered sunlight gave very similar phototoxic protection factors. The phototoxic protection factor (PPF) was defined by the following formula:

$$PPF = \frac{\text{Minimal phototoxic dose in protected skin}}{\text{Minimal phototoxic dose in unprotected skin}}$$

As a result of the confirmation of the validity of the indoor testing, we now feel that when the phototoxic protection factor assay is used with topical methoxalen as the photosensitizer, an appropriately filtered UVA-emitting solar simulator is sufficient. It seems unnecessary to perform outdoor testing to confirm phototoxic protection factors.

In a similar study using oral methoxalen, a similar range of phototoxic protection factors was reported (13). In addition to the evaluation of the minimal phototoxic erythema, these workers also graded pigmentation two weeks after UVA irradiance. They defined a melanogenic protection factor (MPF)(13) and found that both and PPF in methoxalen-photosensitized skin assays gave excellent correlation. In both series of studies, higher protection factors were confirmed using formulations containing the compound Parsol 1789 (butyl methoxydibenzoylmethane) than those containing oxybenzone. The studies performed by Gange et al. (13) used UVA-emitting fluorescent sunlamp tubes. In the studies performed in our own laboratory a filter xenon arc source was used.

It is interesting that similar PPFs were achieved using these different UVA-emitting sources. More convenient UVA sources such as filtered high pressure metal halide lamps give a similar PPF results (Lowe, NJ, unpublished data).

It is likely that different PPFs for the same sunscreen, however, can be obtained from different UV spectrum sources and using photosensitizers with different action spectra from methoxalen. Alternatives include dimethylchlortetracycline (14). These different photosensitizers may result in a shift in action spectra relative to the absorption characteristics of sunscreens to be tested. These important limitations must be borne in mind when interpreting phototoxic protection factors.

Despite these concerns we feel the PPF factor utilizing topical methoxalen as photosensitizer and a broad UVA emitting source is an appropriate means of evaluating UVA sunscreens for the following reasons:

1. Short irradiance times are required
2. Localized skin photosensitization is produced versus generalized skin photosensitization when systemic psoralen is used
3. No systemic toxicity is likely with topical psoralen delivery
4. There is clinical relevance for photoprotection of photosensitized individuals
5. In trained hands this technique is reproducible

IV. SUMMARY OF EVALUATION OF UVA PHOTOPROTECTION

The evaluation of UVA-absorbing sunscreens is a newly emerging area that requires further careful investigation. There are a number of alternative ways of evaluating UVA sunscreens including the use of UVA-induced erythema and immediate pigment darkening in nonphotosensitized individuals. The use of an appropriate photosensitizer such as 8-methoxypsoralen and the establishment of a phototoxic protection factor. It is advisable that UVA emitting sources have a broad range of UVA output to cover both the action spectra of the photosensitized erythema as well as the absorption spectra of the sunscreen to be tested. Suitable UV sources would appear to be appropriately filtered xenon arc or high-pressure metal halide sources. Careful comparative evaluation with other assays should continue in the area of assessment of UVA photoprotecting chemicals.

REFERENCES

1. Staberg, B., Wulf, H. C., Poulsen, T., Klemp, P., and Brodhagen, H. The carcinogenic effect of sequential artificial sunlight + UVA irradiation in hairless mice. Consequences for solarium "therapy." *Arch. Dermatol.,* *119*:641–642 (1983).
2. Paul, B. S. and Parrish, J. A. The interaction of UVA and UVB in the production of threshold erythema. *J. Invest. Dermatol., 78*:371–374 (1982).
3. Gilchrest, B. A., Soter, N. A., Hawk, J. L. M., Barr, R. M., Black, A. K., Hensby, C. N., Mallet, A. I., Greaves, N. W., and Parrish, J. A. Histologic changes associated with ultraviolet A-induced erythema in normal human skin. *J. Am. Acad. Dermatol., 9*:213–219 (1983).
4. Gschnait, F., Schwarz, T., and Ladich, I. Treatment of polymorphous light eruption. *Arch. Dermatol. Res., 275*:379–382 (1983).
5. McFadden, N. UVA sensitivity and topical photoprotection in polymorphous light eruption. *Photodermatology, 1*:76–78 (1984).
6. Diffey, B. L. and Farr, P. M. An evaluation of sunscreens in patients with broad action-spectrum photosensitivity. *Br. J. Dermatol., 112*:83–86 (1985).
7. Sunscreen products for over-the-counter use. *Fed. Reg., 43*:28206–28269 (1978).
8. Lowe, N. J., Dromgoole, S. H., Sefton, J., Bourget, T., and Weingarten, D. Indoor and outdoor efficacy testing of a broad-spectrum sunscreen against ultraviolet A radiation in psoralen-sensitized subjects. *J. Am. Acad. Dermatol., 17*:224–230 (1987).
9. Lowe, N. J., Weingarten, D., and Wortzman, M. Sunscreens and photo-testing. *Clin. Dermatol., 6*:40–49 (1988).
10. Mutzhas, M. F., Holzle, E., Hofmann, C., and Plewig, G. A new apparatus with high radiation energy between 320–460 nm: physical description and dermatological applications. *J. Invest. Dermatol., 76*:42–47 (1981).

11. Ruger, R., Holzle, E., Plewig, G., and Galosi, A. In-vivo-UVA-tests: erythema, pigmentation, phototoxicity, *Skin Models* (Marks R, Plewig G, eds.), Springer-Verlag, Berlin (1986), pp. 147–154.
12. Kaidbey, K. and Gange, R. W. Comparison of methods for assessing photoprotection against ultraviolet A in vivo. *J. Am. Acad. Dermatol.*, *16*:346–353 (1987).
13. Gange, R. W., Soparkar, A., Matzinger, E., Dromgoole, S. H., Sefton, J., and DeGryse, R. Efficacy of a sunscreen containing butyl methoxydibenzoylmethane against ultraviolet A radiation in photosensitized subjects. *J. Am. Acad. Dermatol.*, *15*:494–499 (1986).
14. Dahlen, R. F., Shapiro, S. I., Berry, C. Z., and Schreiber, M. M. A method for evaluating sunscreen protection from long-wave ultraviolet. *J. Invest. Dermatol.*, *55*:164–169 (1970).

15
UVA Protection Factors

JOSEPH W. STANFIELD, STEWART B. SISKIN, and LINCOLN KROCHMAL
Bristol-Myers Squibb Company, Buffalo, New York

I. INTRODUCTION

The total irradiance from the ultraviolet portion of sunlight at 40° north latitude at noon in June is on the order of 5 mW/cm^2, including both direct sunlight and the scattered energy reflected from the sky (1). The major portion of solar ultraviolet radiation is from the UVA region (320–400 nm). A lesser portion, about 3–4%, is from the UVB region (290–320 nm), while terrestrial solar radiation from wavelengths below 290 nm is negligible (2). Since radiation with shorter wavelengths is more readily scattered by constituents of the atmosphere than UVA radiation with longer wavelengths, total UVB is more variable with cloud cover and sun angle than UVA. At Copenhagen (55° north latitude) in winter, the intensity of direct UVA radiation is 10% of that in summer, whereas winter UVB is only 1% of that in summer. Even with 83% cloud cover, the UVA intensity is reduced by only about one-half (2).

The possible daily dose of solar UV in Philadelphia (40° north latitude) is up to 15 minimal erythema doses (MEDs) from UVB and approximately 3 MEDs from UVA (3). Although UVA is only about one-thousandth as effective in producing erythema as UVB (4), UVA alone has been shown to produce many of the potentially deleterious effects of ultraviolet radiation, including pyrimidine dimer formation (5), inhibition of DNA synthesis (6), depletion of epidermal Langerhans cells (7), and elastic fiber damage (8). In addition, UVA wavelengths are responsible for pathologic reactions such as polymorphous light eruption and solar urticaria (4), and a number of phototoxic drug reactions (9,10). Currently marketed sunscreen products with sun protection factors (SPFs) greater than 30 protect against sunburn for a full day's exposure at virtually any location on earth, assuming a sufficient amount is applied, the product is not removed by swimming, perspiration, or physical contact, and assuming no photochemical degradation or cutaneous absorption of active ingredients. However, there is concern among dermatologists that cosmetically acceptable sunscreen products provide incomplete protection in the UVA region (11) and may permit greater exposure to suberythemogenic doses of UV than possible without their use (12). According to Parrish et al. (13), essentially any UV dose produces some cell injury.

The answer to this problem lies in the formulation of improved sunscreen products which provide greater protection in the UVA region. For individuals with skin types I and II (see Table 1), a UVA protection factor of 3–6 would be required for all-day protection against UVA erythema. Since the UVA region is adjacent to the visible light region, increasing the longwave absorbance of sunscreens runs the risk of producing unacceptably opaque or colored products (14), which could be rejected by consumers. Thus the development of UVA protective sunscreens presents a challenge both for the synthetic chemist and the product formulator.

Another challenge faced by sunscreen manufacturers is the measurement and validation of UVA protection. One convenient measure of UV effect on skin is erythema. Since the erythemal effectiveness spectrum closely parallels the spectra for pyrimidine dimer formation and inhibition of DNA synthesis, at least for wavelengths longer than 290 nm (12,15), UV-induced erythema is a highly relevant endpoint for assessing sunscreen protection. However, the assessment of UVA sunscreen protection using the erythemal response requires much higher irradiance levels than previously available or much longer exposure times than required for SPF measurements as currently practiced, since UVA erythema requires 1000 times as much energy as UVB erythema (16).

The following sections present a review of methods for assessing UVA protection and a proposed protocol for measuring UVA protection using the normal erythemal response of sun-sensitive individuals (skin types I and II). We have

Table 1 Classification of Skin Types

Type	Reported reaction to first sun exposure in summer (15–30 min)
I	Always burn, never tan
II	Usually burn, tan with difficulty
III	Sometimes mild burn, tan about average
IV	Rarely burn, tan easily

Source: Adapted from Ref. 17.

coined the term APF to denote the index of UVA protection measured in this manner. APF is analogous in all respects to SPF, which is primarily an index of UVB protection.

II. CURRENT METHODS FOR ASSESSING UVA PROTECTION

A. Erythema in Unsensitized Subjects

The ideal evaluation of sunscreen protection from solar UVA for the general population would be to measure lifetime solar damage to the skin in normal, unsensitized subjects with and without the sunscreen. Since this is obviously impractical, a few compromises are necessary. Sunlight can be replaced with UV radiation from a xenon arc solar simulator, which produces a spectrum representative of the wide range of possible solar spectra, but with an intensity 10–100 times greater. The variety of forms of possible solar damage can be replaced with a single conveniently measured endpoint: erythema. Although these compromises make laboratory assessment of sunscreens far removed from the real situation it is intended to simulate, this artificial set of conditions would represent the best practical means for evaluating the UVA protection of sunscreens.

Typical xenon arc solar simulators deliver UVB energy doses (mJ/cm^2) at rates on the order of 1 mW/cm^2 (irradiance). Since typical MEDs for UVB for skin types I and II are about 20 mJ/cm^2 (17), the time required to produce the MED is on the order of 20 seconds. Thus for a sunscreen with an SPF of 15, a typical exposure series of 9.6, 12, 15, 18.75, and 23.4 MEDs, as prescribed by the FDA proposed monograph (18), would require a total exposure time for each subject of approximately 30 minutes. For a sunscreen with an expected UVA protection factor of 3, the analogous exposure series would be 1.9, 2.4, 3, 3.75, and 4.7 MEDs of UVA, using the prescribed five exposures with doses increasing by 25%. With the UVB portion of the spectrum removed by a WG345 UVB cutoff filter and the remaining UVA irradiance typically about 20 mW/cm^2, the total exposure time for the same subject with a UVA MED of 20 J/cm^2, 1000-fold greater than that for UVB (19), would be over 4 hours, since it takes 1000 seconds to deliver 20 J/cm^2 using an irradiance of 20 mw/cm^2. This exposure time is prohibitive, especially since it is desirable to evaluate one or more test formulations and a control with a known protection factor, simultaneously in each subject. Thus the use of the unsensitized erythema response for evaluating UVA protection presents formidable problems.

B. Psoralen Sensitization

An alternate approach to the evaluation of UVA protection is to sensitize subjects to UVA using oral or topical 8-methoxypsoralen (8-MOP), which lowers the threshold erythema dose by a factor of almost 100 (20), producing acceptable exposure times. With 8-MOP sensitization, erythema manifests optimally at 72 hours and its threshold dose is called the minimal phototoxic dose (MPD). Since the ability of longer wavelengths to produce erythema is enhanced for 8-MOP-sensitized subjects, their response is not typical of that of normal subjects exposed to sunlight (3,21). A sunscreen product with maximum absorbance in the longer wavelengths may yield a higher UVA protection factor than a product with a peak absorbance at shorter wavelengths; the product with a peak absorbance at the shorter wavelengths might be more photoprotective for normal subjects in sunlight. Moreover, there are potential side effects associated with the use of psoralens, such as enhanced sun sensitivity and persistent spots of pigmentation (3). Similar problems are encountered with the use of other chemical photosensitizers such as anthracene. These disadvantages make the use of chemical photosensitizers undesirable.

C. Pigmentation Responses

Other possible endpoints for evaluating UVA protection include immediate and delayed pigmentation. Immediate pigment darkening (IPD) is an oxygen-dependent photochemical reaction of melanin or its precursors in existing melanosomes (22,23). The response is a gray-brown pigmentation which appears during or immediately after irradiation and fades over a period ranging from a few minutes to a few hours (24). The threshold dose is greater than $20 \, J/cm^2$ in subjects with skin type II, but about $3 \, J/cm^2$ in subjects with skin type III (23). For UVA doses greater than approximately $18 \, J/cm^2$, the reaction fades only slightly, or not at all, and persists past the appearance of delayed tanning. IPD is most easily elicited in subjects with skin types III and IV. It is minimal or absent in types I and II and difficult to discern in types IV and V due to pre-existing pigmentation (22). Wavelengths which are capable of producing IPD range from UVB through visible radiation (25), however the most effective wavelengths are 320–340 nm (26). The low threshold doses required (exposure times of less than 3 minutes) and the immediacy of results make IPD attractive for measuring UVA protection. However, the high effectiveness of longer wavelengths in producing IPD, coupled with low UV absorbance of sunscreen products in that region, may cause underestimation of sunscreen protection against photodamage from shorter wavelengths.

Delayed pigmentation (tanning) represents proliferation of melanocytes and increased production of melanosomes (26). Wavelengths in the UVB region are most effective for producing tanning as well as erythema (12,26). However, repeated suberythemogenic doses of UVA readily produce tanning (13). According to Kagetsu et al. (27) the mean threshold dose for 20 subjects with skin types I, II, and III was $19–33 \, J/cm^2$ for UVA-induced tanning with distinct borders, observed at 24 hours. Approximately the same UVA doses were required for the same degree of tanning observed at 48 hours and 7 days. An almost twofold difference was observed for the threshold tanning dose when it was administered at 5 mW/cm^2 instead of 50 mW/cm^2. Thus dose reciprocity was not conserved.

Pigmentation responses are most apparent in those individuals who require sunscreen protection least and are difficult to elicit in those most susceptible to solar injury. This militates against utilization of these endpoints for evaluating UVA protection.

III. USE OF MODIFIED SOLAR SIMULATORS

A. Optical Concentration of Irradiance

An approach which might permit utilization of the normal erythema response for evaluating UVA protection is to employ a solar simulator capable of much higher UVA irradiance values than the typical 20 mW/cm^2. For a 2500 W xenon arc solar simulator, we have used a quartz lens to focus the 8 cm diameter beam to a 1.5 cm diameter spot, achieving UVA irradiance values as high as 250 mW/cm^2. UVB wavelengths were removed using a 2 mm Schott WG345 filter. The unwanted increase in visible and infrared energy was removed using a black glass filter (Schott UG-11) and 10 cm light path circulating water filter. Since the black glass filter absorbs sufficient energy to cause fracturing due to thermal stresses, it was placed within the circulating water filter to provide cooling. The irradiance was maintained at 100 mW/cm^2 by varying the lamp input voltage and placing a 1 mm stainless steel wire mesh screen in the path of the beam. All measurable spectral irradiance ($>10^{-10}$ w/cm^2/nm) was from UVA wavelengths.* The lamp spectrum is shown in Figure 1.

B. Dose Reciprocity

A potentially serious problem with the use of high irradiance values is the possible breakdown of dose reciprocity, which could invalidate assessments of UVA photoprotection. Kagetsu et al. (27) observed that the MED (mean for 6 subjects) was 53 J/cm^2 for a UVA irradiance of 50 mW/cm^2 and 68 J/cm^2 for an irradiance of 5 mW/cm^2. This difference was statistically significant. However, its potential clinical significance in the evaluation of sunscreen products appears marginal, since it represents only a 22% reduction in MED. In our own laboratory we have demonstrated reciprocity for MED and UVA protection factor for irradiance values of 50 and 100 mW/cm^2 in normal, sun-sensitive subjects, evaluated approximately 24 hours after exposure (19). Diffey et al. have shown that

---

*Optronic Model 742 Spectroradiometer, Optronic Laboratories, Orlando, FL.

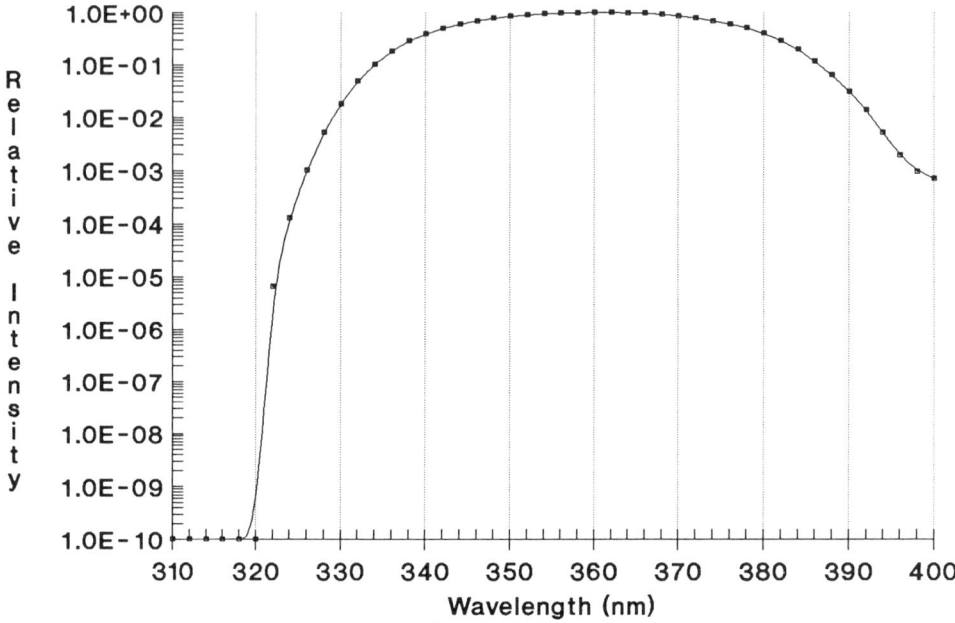

Figure 1   Spectral irradiance of solar simulator.

intensity of erythema at 24 hours was not dependent on dose rate (28). However, the equivalence of UVA protection factor measured using an irradiance of 100 mW/cm² to that for outdoor solar radiation has not been demonstrated conclusively.

C. Pain Threshold

Diffey reported that subjects experienced pain at irradiances higher than 110 mW/cm² (28). In our laboratory we have recorded instances of mild discomfort described as an itching, prickling sensation for irradiance values in excess of 180 mW/cm². Pain during irradiation is attributed to a thermal effect in which energy is delivered to a shallow layer of the skin at a faster rate than it can be dissipated, resulting in a temperature increase. Using a surface temperature probe, we observed a skin temperature increase of 4°C which remained stable during prolonged irradiation at 100 mW/cm². A temperature increase of approximately 9°C would be required for the pain threshold to be reached. Reports of discomfort for irradiance values of 100 mW/cm^2 or less have been rare.

D. Radiometry

Several investigators (11,16,27) have utilized photodiode UVA probes* with peak spectral responses in the vicinity of 360 nm for measuring UVA irradiance. These investigators have reported UVA MEDs of about 40 J/cm^2. We have used a similar probe, but its peak response is at 350 nm. This may account for the fact that our observed MED for UVA is about 20 J/cm^2. Paul and Parrish (5) reported MED values comparable to our own for irradiance measured with a similar probe. For standardization of UV sources it would be preferable to report irradiance values as the irradiance integrated over a stated range of the lamp spectrum obtained using a high-precision spectroradiometer. However even this alternative presents problems in determining absolute irradiance values due to variables in beam geometry, distance from the source, and instrument input optics.

IV. COMPARATIVE STUDIES OF PHOTOPROTECTION

Kaidbey and Gange (4) studied the UVA protection of three sunscreens using erythema and pigmentation in unsensitized subjects and in subjects photosensitized with topical 8-MOP or anthracene. For Parsol 1789† (2%) and Eusolex 8020‡ (2%) mean phototoxic protection factors of approximately 3 were obtained for sensitized skin and protection factors of approximately 1.8 and 1.4, respectively, were obtained at 24 hour evaluations of erythema in unsensitized subjects. Using immediate pigment darkening and delayed tanning at 7 days, protection factors ranged from 1.6 to 1.8. For oxybenzone (3%) phototoxic protection factors of 2.0 and 1.8 were obtained for 8-MOP and anthracene sensitization, respectively, and in unsensitized subjects protection factors were 1.6 for 24 hour erythema and 1.3 to 1.4 for immediate and delayed tanning. They concluded that sensitized subjects yielded higher protection factors than unsensitized subjects for Parsol 1789 and Eusolex 8020 but not for oxybenzone.

Gange et al. (11) evaluated Parsol 1789 (3%) in skin sensitized with oral 8-MOP and obtained mean phototoxic protection factors of 3.3 for 48 hour evaluations and 4.1 for 72 hour evaluations. The mean melanogenic protection factor at 12–18 days was 3.7.

---

*International Light Company, Newburyport, MA.
†t-butylmethoxydibenzoyl methane.
‡4-isopropyl-dibenzoyl methane.

Using our modified solar simulator, we have assessed the UVA protection factor of a research sunscreen formulation containing oxybenzone (6%). In subjects with skin type II, using 24 hour evaluations of erythema, the mean protection factor was 3.2 (19). Lowe obtained a phototoxic protection factor of 3.1 for the same formulation using 72 hour evaluations of erythema in subjects sensitized with topical 8-MOP and a conventional solar simulator (20).

From the foregoing it appears that evaluations in unsensitized subjects yield lower protection factors than those in sensitized subjects for Parsol 1789 and Eusolex 8020, but similar results for oxybenzone.

V. PROPOSED PROTOCOL

A. Light Source

The light source is a xenon arc lamp with a 2 mm Schott WG345 filter for removal of UVB and a water filter and black glass (UG-11) filter for removal of visible and infrared. The irradiance should not exceed 100 mW/cm^2 and the spectral irradiance from UVB wavelengths should be at least five orders of magnitude below the irradiance from UVA wavelengths. The beam should be uniform within ± 25% and at least 1 cm in diameter.

B. Subjects

Subjects should be of skin type I or II to minimize MED times and preclude delayed tanning which obscures erythema, and should be free from any dermatologic condition or use of any potentially photosensitizing or anti-inflammatory drug. The midback area should be free from any sunburn, tan, lesions, or hair which might interfere with the administration of treatment or evaluation of responses.

C. Initial MED Determination

Within 1 week before the test the subject's UVA MED is determined by administering at least three UVA exposures to the midback in exposure increments of 25%. The MED is the lowest UVA dose which produces erythema with distinct borders 24 ± 2 hours later and is used to establish subsequent UVA exposures.

D. Test Products

Test products should include a standard (control) with a known protection factor, such as a 6% solution of oxybenzone (APF of approximately 3). Test products should be applied at a dosage of 2 μl/cm^2 using a gloved finger to an area of at least 50 cm^2 and allowed to dry for at least 15 minutes. Products should be applied with the subject in the same position as will be used for UVA exposures. The number of test products to be evaluated will be determined by the MED time and the expected product APFs. In general the total time required for all UVA exposures should not exceed 2 hours.

E. UVA Exposures

At least three UVA exposures should be administered in 25% increments with the expected product APF times the initial MED used as the center site. Exposed sites should be marked using an indelible pen. An unprotected site should receive the same number of exposures to permit determination of the final MED.

F. APF Evaluations

At 24 ± 2 hours after beginning exposures, subjects should be evaluated as was done for the initial MED. Lighting should be consistent and directed to avoid producing shadows. The evaluator should be blinded with respect to the identity of treatments and UV exposures. Any exposure series which yields definite erythema at all sites or no erythema at any site should be repeated with UV exposures adjusted to lower or higher values. APF is the ratio of protected to final unprotected MED.

G. Calculation of APF

Product APF should be calculated as the mean for a panel of at least 20 subjects with a standard error of 5% or less, as is done with SPF.

VI. CONCLUSION

A proposed protocol has been presented for determining the UVA protection factor, denoted APF, for sunscreen products. We believe the use of xenon arc solar simulators with high irradiance rates and unsensitized subjects with skin types I and II can permit meaningful assessments of the protectiveness of sunscreens in the UVA region as is currently accomplished for the full solar spectrum through SPF determinations. Erythema in unsensitized subjects is considered a more relevant index of potential solar damage than 8-MOP phototoxicity or immediate or delayed pigmentation. Although the question of UVA dose reciprocity is not fully resolved, MEDs for high irradiance rates are similar to those reported for much lower irradiance values.

An additional index of sunscreen protection can serve as a goal for manufacturers and can effectively guide physicians and consumers in selecting the maximum available protection against the damaging effects of sunlight.

REFERENCES

1. Berger, D. S. Specification and design of solar ultraviolet simulators. *J. Invest. Dermatol.*, *53*:192–199 (1969).
2. Gilchrest, B. A., Soter, N., Hawk, J. L. M., Barr, R., Black, A., Hensby, C., Mallet, A., Greaves, M., and Parrish, J. Histologic changes associated with ultraviolet A-induced erythema in normal human skin. *J. Am. Acad. Dermatol.*, *9*:213–219 (1983).
3. Kromann, N., Wulf, H. C., Eriksen, P., and Brodthagen, H. Relative ultraviolet spectral intensity of direct solar radiation, sky radiation and surface reflections. *Photodermatology*, *3*:73–82 (1986).
4. Kaidbey, K. and Gange, R. W. Comparison of methods for assessing photoprotection against ultraviolet A in vivo. *J. Am. Acad. Dermatol.*, *16*:346–353 (1987).
5. Paul, B. S. and Parrish, J. A. The interaction of UVA and UVB in the production of threshold erythema. *J. Invest. Dermatol.*, *79*:371–374 (1982).
6. Freeman, S. E., Gange, R. W., Sutherland, J. C., and Sutherland, B. M. Pyrimidine dimer formation in human skin. *Photochem. Photobiol.*, *46*:202–212 (1987).
7. Chew, S., DeLeo, V., and Harber, L. Longwave ultraviolet radiation (UVA)-induced alteration of epidermal DNA synthesis. *Photochem. Photobiol.*, *47*:383–389 (1988).
8. Kligman, L., Akin, F., and Kligman, A. The contributions of UVA and UVB to connective tissue damage in hairless mice. *J. Invest. Dermatol.*, *84*:272–276 (1985).
9. Addo, H., Ferguson, J., and Frain-Bell, W. Thiazide-induced photosensitivity: a study of 33 subjects. *Br. Dermatol.*, *116*:749–760 (1987).
10. Fujita, H. and Matsuo, I. UVA induced DNA nicking activities of skin photosensitive drugs: phenothiazines, benzothiadiazines and afloqualone. *Chem. Biol. Interact.*, *66*:27–36 (1988).
11. Gange, R., Soparkar, A., Matzinger, E., Dromgoole, S., Sefton, J., and DeGryse, R. Efficacy of a sunscreen containing butyl methoxydibenzoylmethane against ultraviolet A radiation in photosensitized subjects. *J. Am. Acad. Sci.*, *15*:494–499 (1986).
12. Parrish, J., Jaenicke, K. F., and Anderson, R. R. Erythema and melanogenesis action spectra of normal human skin. *Photochem. Photobiol.*, *36*:187–191 (1982).
13. Parrish, J., Zaynoun, S., and Anderson, R. Cumulative effects of repeated subthreshold doses of ultraviolet radiation. *J. Invest. Dermatol.*, *76*:356–358 (1981).
14. Johnson, J. A. and Fusaro, R. M. Protection against long ultraviolet radiation: topical browning agents and a new outlook. *Dermatologica*, *175*:53–57 (1987).
15. Kaidbey, K. Wavelength dependence for DNA synthesis inhibition in hairless mouse epidermis. *Photodermatology*, *5*:65–70 (1988).

16. Lowe, N. J., Weingarten, D., and Wortzman, M. Sunscreens and photo-testing. *Clin. Dermatol., 6*:40–49 (1988).
17. Fitzpatrick, T. The validity and practicality of sun-reactive skin types I through IV. *Arch. Dermatol., 124*:869–871 (1988).
18. Department of Health, Education and Welfare. Sunscreen drug products for over-the-counter human use. *Fed. Reg., 43*:38206–38269 (1978).
19. Stanfield, J. W., Feldt, P. A., Csortan, E. S., and Krochmal, L. UVA sunscreen evaluations in normal subjects. *J. Am. Acad. Dermatol., 20*:744-748 (1989).
20. Study DE116-004-001. Bristol-Myers Squibb Pharmaceutical Research and Development, Buffalo, NY (1988).
21. Cripps, D., Lowe, N., and Lerner, A. Action spectra of topical psoralens: a re-evaluation. *Br. J. Dermatol., 107*:77–82 (1982).
22. Beitner, H. Immediate pigment-darkening reaction. *Photodermatology, 5*: 96–100 (1988).
23. Beitner, H. and Wennersten, G. A qualitative and quantitative transmission electromicroscopic study of the immediate pigment darkening reaction. *Photodermatology, 2*:273–278 (1985).
24. Kaidbey, K. H. and Kligman, A. M. The acute effects of long-wave ultraviolet radiation on human skin. *J. Invest. Dermatol., 72*:253–256 (1978).
25. Pathak, M. A., Riley, F. C., and Fitzpatrick, T. B. Melanogenesis in human skin following exposure to long-wave ultraviolet and visible light. *J. Invest. Dermatol., 39*:435–443 (1962).
26. Pathak, M. Activation of the melanocyte system by ultraviolet radiation and cell transformation. *Ann. NY Acad. Sci., 453*:328–339 (1985).
27. Kagetsu, N., Gange, R. W., and Parrish, J. A. UVA-induced erythema, pigmentation, and skin surface temperature changes are irradiance dependent. *J. Invest. Dermatol., 85*:445–447 (1985).
28. Diffey, B. L., Farr, P. M., and Oakley, A. M. Quantitative studies on UVA-induced erythema in human skin. *Br. J. Dermatol., 117*:57–66 (1987).

SELECTED SUNSCREEN FORMULATIONS AVAILABLE
IN THE UNITED STATES

Trade Name and (Manufacturer)	SPF
SPF Higher Than 15	
Bain de Soleil (Bain de Soleil)	30
Block Out (Carter Products)	30
Cancer Garde (Eclipse Labs)	30
Coppertone (Plough)	30
PreSun for Kids (Westwood)	39
PreSun 29 (Westwood)	29
Solbar (Person and Covey)	50
Sundown (Johnson & Johnson)	20
Sundown (Johnson & Johnson)	30
Supershade (Plough)	44
T/I Screen (T/I Pharmaceuticals)	30
Ultrashade (Plough)	23
SPF of 15	
Block Out (Carter Products)	15
Coppertone (Plough)	15
Neutrogena Facial Sunscreen (Neutrogena)	15
Photoplex (Herbert Labs)	15
PreSun (Westwood)	15
Sundown (Johnson & Johnson)	15
Supershade (Plough)	15
Total Eclipse (Eclipse Labs)	15
Water Babies (Plough)	15
Lipstick Sunscreens	
Clinique Paba-Free (Clinique)	22
Neutrogena Lip Moisturizer (Neutrogena)	15
Physician's Formula Sunshield (Physician's Formula)	15
Presun Protector (Westwood)	15
Sundown Sunblock (Johnson & Johnson)	20
T/I Sunscreen Non-Paba (T/I Pharmaceuticals)	15
Total Eclipse (Eclipse Labs)	15

Index

About the Editor

NICHOLAS J. LOWE is Medical Director of the Skin Research Foundation of California, Director of the Southern California Dermatology and Psoriasis Center, Santa Monica, and Clinical Professor of Dermatology, UCLA School of Medicine, Los Angeles, California. A recipient of numerous awards from the American Academy of Dermatology, Dr. Lowe serves on the editorial boards of several dermatologic journals and has published over 200 articles. A Diplomate of the American Board of Dermatology and Fellow of the American Academy of Dermatology, he received the **M.D.** degree (1968) from the University of Liverpool, England.